The Super Easy UK 5-Ingredient Low-Carb Recipe Book

300+ Effortless and Delicious Recipes
for Busy People Eager to Embrace a Healthy Low-Carb Lifestyle
I 28-Day Meal Plan Included I

Amanda Lloyd

TABLE OF CONTENTS

Introduction

This is a practical guide on the low-carb diet.

We will show you why this type of diet is so effective, what its main benefits are, what the best tips and mistakes to avoid, ensuring that you can get back in shape.

There will be a totally practical part in which we will show you 300 recipes divided into various categories. These recipes, as well as being delicious will also be quite easy to make. It is, in fact, a recipe with 5 ingredients and rather fast, all based on the low-carb style.

There will be a 4-week meal plan too, in which you will also be explained how to set up your daily meals. Having said that, we want you to introduce to what a low-carb diet is.

The low-carb diet is not just a choice that is very trendy nowadays, but a real lifestyle that allows you to lose weight constantly and, above all, safely. In fact, there are many low-carb diets that are very fashionable: from the paleo to the well-known ketogenic diet, to the Atkins', all of which have a common point, namely the very low-carbohydrate intake. This drop-in carbohydrate intake also works in favour of other macronutrients, such as fats or proteins.

What therefore unites all these various dietary regimes is precisely the fact of being "low" with a low-carb content, or carbohydrates.

This is because carbohydrates, along with fat, are our main source of energy. And as part of a low-carb diet program, carbohydrates are consciously reduced to lose body fat. But how do carbohydrates, according to this current of thought, affect weight and body fat? Carbohydrates have a significant impact on body fat percentage when the body obtains more than it requires. Specifically, in fact, excess carbohydrates are stored in the form of fat reserves for any moment of need. And in the long run, these fat stores are accumulating more and more. We must also consider the fact that sugars, especially simple ones, tend to be addictive, causing their intake to grow exponentially.

In any case, low-carb diets begin to make their way in this period and, thanks to their effective contribution in the loss of excess body weight, they become the prevailing and among the most used diets.

How does this type of diet work?

Low-carb diets limit carbohydrate intake to fewer than 100 gr per day, split evenly between simple and complex carbohydrates. The maximum carb limit must never be exceeded.

And it is the low-carbohydrate intake that will lead to the loss of body fat. In practice, the principle of this diet is the fact that the body reacts to the lack of carbohydrates by affecting the reserves in order to have enough energy. These energy reserves are represented by glycogen (the glucose "stored" in the liver) which is attacked first and, subsequently, the lipids, or the reserve fat accumulated in the body in a localized way, will be attacked.

As for the distribution of the other energetic macronutrients, it varies according to the current of thought.

As we have already said above, there are different types of low-carb diets, but even if they have one point in common, that is the lower intake of carbohydrates, they differ, however, based on the distribution of macronutrients.

Some claim that a low-carb diet should be high in fat (thus a hyper lipid type diet) while maintaining a similar quantity of proteins, resulting in a nutritional breakdown that looks like this:

✓ 50-60% of lipids

✓ 20-30% of proteins

Others, on the other hand, believe that it is essential to almost totally eliminate foods that contain carbohydrates, freely increasing protein intake (also in view of preserving lean mass) and thus determining a division more similar to this:

✓ 30% of lipids

✓ 60% proteins

The low-carb diet is therefore effective because it can be suitable for all those who want to burn fat and define their body.

This is because a low-body type of diet also aims at preserving lean mass (thanks to the protein supply) and body recomposition.

But its greatest effectiveness lies in the loss of body fat. Weight loss will inevitably be caused by reducing the pockets of excess fat in the body.

Benefits of low-carb diet

After explaining what the low-carb diet is, how it works and why it is effective, let's deepen the concept of the effectiveness of this diet, listing its benefits.

So, what are the main benefits of a low-carb diet? Let's see them together:

Reduces your appetite

With a low-carb diet, you will have greater control of your appetite and hunger cravings.

It is well known that the intake of sugar contributes to addiction. This is because the continuous intake of sugar creates insulin peaks. Thanks to the low sugar intake, you will no longer have so-called insulin peaks. Consequently, not only will the sense of hunger decrease, but, on the other hand, that of satiety will increase. In addition to all this, you will have greater control over nervous hunger and sudden cravings for sweets. There is also the fact that low-carb diets are based on foods rich in protein, and it is well known that protein is the nutrient that is digested more slowly. To put it another way, protein keep you full for a long period. Those who are full are less likely to seek out food or sweets.

Effective for weight loss

There will be a general weight loss. Thanks to a low-carb diet, it will be easier to lose weight in general and, especially initially, faster. This is because, as we explained in the introduction, when there is a lack of glucose, the reserves of fat will be affected to ensure that the body procures the energy necessary for itself to survive. In addition to all this, a low-carb diet will lead to a marked improvement in the conditions of the metabolism. Thanks to the fact that the sugar / fat reserve ratio is reset, the metabolism will also benefit and return to its normal functions.

Promotes fat loss from your abdominal cavity firstly

A low-carb diet, as well as allowing a general and widespread weight loss, will also allow you to affect firstly the fat abdominal stores which are so dangerous for health, especially for that of the heart. According to research comparing low-carb and low fat diets, low-carb eating reduces fat in the abdomen and around the organs, including the liver. This shows that part of the fat lost as a result of a low-carbohydrate diet is harmful belly fat.

Helps you lower triglycerides

Low-carb diets cause triglyceride levels to drop, according to numerous studies. The results are constant and striking.

A lowering of blood triglycerides has even been called "the hallmark of a low-carb diet," and many doctors are now recommending reducing carbs as the first line of defence against high triglyceride levels. In addition, many doctors who recommend low-carbohydrate diets to their patients use blood triglycerides as a marker to tell if the patient is following the diet faithfully.

Increases levels of good HDL cholesterol

In addition to helping to reduce bad cholesterol levels and triglycerides in the blood, a low-carb diet could really help you to increase levels of good cholesterol (HDL).

HDL cholesterol appears to protect against heart disease; it becomes a risk factor for heart disease if it is low, so eating low carb can help in that regard as well.

Helps you lower blood pressure

Excess weight loss has a direct effect of lowering blood pressure when following a low-carb diet. Increased blood pressure is not something you should be concerned about or perceive, but it is a condition that, if left untreated, can lead to a variety of health issues.

By avoiding refined sweets, bread, carbonated beverages, convenience foods, and fast food, you will not only lower your carbohydrate intake, but also your salt intake, which is abundantly added to all of these meals and is one of the main causes of hypertension.

Helps you reduce blood sugar and insulin levels, and maintain lower the risk of type 2 diabetes

It has shown that a low-carb diet could bring advantages in the treatment of metabolic diseases such as diabetes and insulin resistance: thanks to the reduced intake of carbohydrates and therefore the absence of blood sugar or insulin peaks, this type of diet can really help in the prevention and treatment of diabetes or pathologies related to the dysfunction of the insulin level in the blood. The stabilization of the glycaemic rate, thanks to the low sugar intake could reduce insulin levels too.

Fights the metabolic syndrome

Metabolic syndrome is a syndrome that has been linked to an increased risk of diabetes and heart disease. In reality, the metabolic syndrome is characterized by a number of symptoms, including:

- ✓ Abdominal obesity.
- ✓ Blood pressure that is too high.
- ✓ High blood sugar levels after a fast.
- ✓ Triglycerides that aren't typical.

Low HDL cholesterol levels, sometimes known as "good cholesterol".

A low-carb diet, on the other hand, has been shown to be quite beneficial in addressing all five of these symptoms in trials.

It is therapeutic for some brain disorders

A low-carbohydrate diet has also been demonstrated to increase brain performance.

Ketones, which are produced as a result of a low-carbohydrate diet, have been proven to be one of the best sources of fuel for your brain, as well as neuroprotective antioxidants.

Numerous studies have confirmed its usefulness in preventing disorders including Alzheimer's and epilepsy.

7 mistakes to avoid on a low-carb diet

Now that we know all the amazing benefits of a low-carb diet, we would like to show you some mistakes to avoid when deciding to take this dietary path.

So, let's see together what the most common mistakes are and how to avoid them:

Focus on carbs only

The wrong thing to do is to be obsessed with carbs.

It is okay that it is a question of lowering the amount of daily carbohydrates to which we may be used to, but our attention must not be focused only on them.

There are other macronutrients such as proteins and fats that are equally fundamental and that we need to face not only the diet but also the day.

These macronutrients must be chosen for excellent quality and contribute to our daily needs. So, just be fixated on carbs and focus our attention on the quality of fats and proteins.

Avoiding vegetable and fibres

There is nothing more wrong than not taking vegetables and fibres. Vegetables, especially those with green leaves, are very rich in fibre. Fibres are essential for the absorption of sugars. The recipes, for example, will also indicate the amount of fibre that you will need to subtract them from the number of carbs and reveal how many are actually in a meal. Therefore, the total carbohydrates are calculated of the fibres. As for vegetables, they are not only important for fibre but also contain essential vitamins for our body. For these fundamental reasons a portion of vegetables should be taken for each meal.

Eating too much dairy

Another mistake for those who want to follow a low-carb dietary path is to eat too much dairy. Even if these are low-carb foods, they are very rich in fat. In certain settings or at quantities higher than those recommended by professionals, several of the compounds found in milk and derivatives can be hazardous to one's health. In particular saturated fat and cholesterol or some factors that can worsen some health conditions, such as hypertension or hypercholesterolemia.

Therefore, in a low-carb diet, it is possible to eat dairy products but in limited quantities. Better to prefer other protein sources such as fish or lean meat.

Snacking too much

Eating often may help a slow metabolism to give a boost. However, it is always recommended to limit yourself to two snacks a day (mid-morning and mid-afternoon) so that you don't get super hungry during your main meals. But, if the two snacks are exceeded, there is only the risk of increasing the daily caloric intake and frustrating the efforts of the low-carb diet.

Therefore, limit yourself to having two snacks, because, as we have already stated, it will be the diet itself that will slow down your cravings.

Eating cheat meals

Cheating, it is well known, can really help, especially on a psychological level, to deal with a diet, in particular with such a difficult diet to follow. But obviously it must remain limited to isolated cases. This is because cheating often can only nullify the many sacrifices faced in this diet, because they could compromise ketosis and make you overindulge on calories. Moreover, in the first phase of the low-carb diet, cheatings are absolutely forbidden. This is because the first is the attack phase, the one in which several weight should be lost.

Drinking alcohol

Drinking alcohol in general is awful. This is an effective law for everyone. But, in particular, in a low-carb diet, alcoholic beverages must be banned due to the intake of unnecessary sugars. Sugars that are not foreseen in a diet like that. Not to mention all the damage done to health, liver, and heart conditions.

Drinking too much coffee

Even if coffee is considered a metabolism booster and a hunger cruncher, you shouldn't overdo it. This is because high blood pressure causes worry, nervousness, and a quick heartbeat. Caffeine stimulates the central nervous system, which causes an increase in the release of adrenaline, making you nervous or afraid. A situation of stressing out can lead to eating more, so we advise you not to overdo it with coffees. In addition to the health problems mentioned, there is no need to stress further in an already restrictive diet. Limit yourself to one coffee a day, strictly unsweetened.

5 tips for embracing a perfect low-carb lifestyle

After showing you, which mistakes you should avoid in order to be successful with the low-carb diet, now we will show you 5 very useful tips to deal with this diet at its best.

Thanks for these tips you will embrace a perfect low-

Carb lifestyle.

Have realistic expectations

Expectations boost your confidence in your ability to succeed, and having faith in yourself has tangible advantages. If you feel you can lose weight, you are more likely to succeed; but, if you believe you will fail, you are more likely to fail. One of the most common diet blunders is failing to set goals. Or, even worse, they establish unattainable goals. Goals serve as a road map for the entire weight-loss journey, and the ones you set for yourself early on can have a significant impact on the program's result.

Anyway, when you go on a diet, the important thing is to complete it successfully. You must have realistic expectations.

You must be realistic and have to face:

✓ You have to be aware of the times it will take.

✓ Exercise.

✓ Have patience.

✓ Be constant.

✓ Knowing that there can also be moments of stalemate.

So, set realistic expectations, especially on a low-carb diet. Focus on small achievable changes, so that you can experience feelings of success every week. Take some time to recognize your achievements, no matter how small they may be. In terms of diet and results, start with a modest weight goal: many people have a "ideal" weight in mind that may feel unattainable. Begin with a smaller goal that feels manageable for you. When a goal is met, set a new one and then succeed again.

Stay motivated

A new lifestyle, healthier and more attentive to our body, with weight loss and remodelling of the forms such as low carb, leads as an inevitable consequence such as returning to the right weight for us. This is how the need, without obsessions, to lose a few extra pounds should be experienced, even if, certainly, it is not simple: a strong motivation is needed for the low-carb diet. When dealing with some deprivation, inevitably it is a small sacrifice, which requires commitment, regardless of how much you have to actually lose. Motivation for a diet is fundamental whatever the need that drives us to stay stint or in any case to change eating habits.

Paying attention to nutrition and staying focused on the goal have to do with the confidence and self-esteem you feel in yourself. To keep motivation high for the low-carb diet, make sure that the result you want to achieve is reasonable: do not raise the bar too much by setting too high goals, which you can eventually touch slowly, progressively. Strengthen confidence and self-esteem by thinking about all the successes already achieved in other contexts: rethinking the times you have made it spurs you to maintain the motivation for change. Focus on improvements, however small, and not on setbacks. If when you step on the scale you still do not see a significant drop in the sacrifices you are making, give yourself time and focus on the positive aspects you are experiencing: a sense of greater lightness, more energy, better mood.

Be flexible

Don't be continually obsessed with measuring every single gram of your foods. It is right to measure everything perfectly in the diet, so as not to exceed the calories. But flexibility is also important to stay motivated. This means that even if you have cheated, it does not bring you to give up the diet. You simply have to leave trying to catch up on the next meal and start the next day with the diet. Be flexible is therefore important to achieving your goals.

Sleep enough

Another important thing to remember when on a low-carb diet is the correct amount of rest. This is because sleeping properly is also good for the metabolism itself.

In fact, it has been shown that sleeping too little slows down the metabolism and increases the stimulus of hunger: a combination that will lead us to eat a lot and assimilate and burn less, further straining the metabolism. Sleeping the correct number of hours, no less than 7 for an adult, will help boost the metabolism and deal with the diet.

Don't be stressed out (embrace your new healthy lifestyle serenely)

The best way to deal with any change is to do it with serenity. Change can be scary, especially if we are used to eating a certain way.

Facing this new path with serenity also means not fearing the judgment of others. Starting a diet path means changing your lifestyle and this is a choice for yourself that should not cause any shame.

Don't' be stressed out if there will be difficulties in following this diet. The mistake that most diets have in common lies in an excessive attempt to control food and it is this mental mechanism that spontaneously leads to the same loss of control.

The more something is forbidden, the greater will be the desire to transgress, so it is much more likely that the person who has imposed himself on not giving in to the temptations of food will find himself transgressing in an uncontrolled and boundless way.

The important thing is to know it and be prepared for a few slips, a few cheats.

It is always better to give yourself a small gift of taste and then resume the diet with serenity than constantly feeling frustrated.

Then you can go on without guilt and without devaluing yourself.

300 Low-Carb Recipes

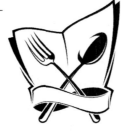

Here you are 300 super easy low-carb recipes.
These are 5 ingredients recipes, easy to make and perfectly suitable for a low-carb diet.

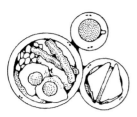

***

Breakfast recipes

Almond pancake

Servings: 4 I Prep time: 10 minutes I Cook time: 5 minutes
Nutrition facts per serving: calories: 200; carbs: 7 gr; protein:12 gr; fat: 8 gr.

Ingredients
✓ 60 gr of almond flour
✓ 2 eggs
✓ 1 tsp of stevia
✓ 60 ml of unsweetened almond milk
✓ 1 tsp of vanilla extract
✓ 1 pinch of backing soda + salt

Directions
➢ Start the recipe by dividing the yolk from the egg white and transfer them to two different bowls.
➢ Add the stevia to the yolk and beat with a whisk.
➢ Add the almond milk too and continue beating.
➢ Then add the almond flour, a pinch of baking soda, a pinch of salt, and vanilla extract.
➢ Stir until you have a smooth mixture.
➢ Then whip the egg whites until stiff and gently incorporate them into the rest of the dough.
➢ Heat a non-stick pan and grease it lightly.
➢ Pour a spoonful of dough for each pancake and wait about a minute.
➢ As soon as the first bubbles form, you can turn them over and continue cooking on the other side.
➢ Continue to cook all the pancakes in this way.
When your pancakes are well done, serve them.

Almond flour and orange microwave cups

Servings: 4 I Prep time: 15 minutes I Cook time: 50 minutes
Nutrition facts per serving: calories 320; carbs: 10 gr; protein: 14 gr; fat: 12 gr.

Ingredients
✓ 4 eggs
✓ 200 gr of almond flour
✓ 1 tbsp of powdered stevia
✓ 4 tbsp of orange juice + 1 tablespoon of grated orange zest
✓ 2 tbsp of melted butter
✓ Backing soda + salt

Directions
➢ First, take the almond flour and put in a bowl together with stevia, a tsp of baking soda and salt.
➢ Combine all the ingredients well.
➢ In a separate bowl, beat the eggs until swollen.
➢ Add the orange juice, melted butter, beaten eggs and orange zest to the almond flour mixture.
➢ Stir until all the ingredients are well blended.
➢ Grease some baking cups with a little margarine.
➢ Spread the smoothing batter into the bowls.
➢ Place in the microwave at high power (800 watts) for about 1 and a half minutes.
➢ This is if you decide to cook one cup at a time.
➢ If you opt, to save time, cook them all together, cook them for about 3 minutes.
➢ Insert a toothpick and if it does not come out dry, bake for another maximum minute until cooked.
➢ Serve the cake just warmed for your breakfast.

Avocado smoked salmon omelette

Servings: 4 I Prep time: 10 minutes I Cook time: 20 minutes
Nutrition facts per serving: calories: 350; carbs:6 gr; protein:22 gr; fat:14 gr.
Ingredients
✓ 6 eggs
✓ 20 ml of olive oil
✓ 120 gr of smoked salmon
✓ 2 avocados
✓ Olive oil

✓   Salt and pepper to taste

Directions
➢   Start with avocados.
➢   Remove the stone from both avocados and wash them.
➢   After that cut them into cubes.
➢   Cut the smoked salmon into little pieces.
➢   Put the eggs in a bowl and beat them vigorously with a fork.
➢   Add a pinch of salt, pepper, then mix the ingredients well.
➢   Add smoked salmon.
➢   Take a non-stick pan.
➢   Heat a little oil and then add a little beaten egg.
➢   Cook for 2 minutes on each side.
➢   Close the omelette, cook for another minute on each side and place it on a serving dish.
➢   Do the same with other omelettes
➢   Place them with cubed avocado in a dish and season with olive oil and a pinch of salt.
➢   Serve salmon omelette with avocado.

Beets scrambled eggs

Servings: 4 I Prep time: 10 minutes I Cook time: 20 minutes
Nutrition facts per serving: calories: 255; carbs: 1 gr; protein: 28 gr; fat: 3 gr.

Ingredients
✓   4 eggs and 2 egg withes
✓   400 gr of beets
✓   3 tbsp of olive oil
✓   2 tsp of chopped chives
✓   Olive oil
✓   Salt and pepper to taste

Directions
➢   First, wash and dry the beets.
➢   Take a non-stick pan and heat the oil.
➢   as soon as it is hot, add the beets and brown it for 5 minutes, seasoning with salt and pepper.
➢   In a dish, lightly beat the eggs and after 5 minutes put the eggs in the pan with the beets.
➢   Stir constantly, so that the eggs do not form an omelette but many separate pieces.
➢   Cook for five minutes and then divide the eggs into 4 serving plates.
➢   Meanwhile, wash and finely chop chives.
➢   Serve the beet eggs sprinkled with chopped chives.

Cheddar spicy frittata

Servings: 4 I Prep time: 15 minutes I Cook time: 30 minutes
Nutrition facts per serving: calories: 190; carbs: 2 gr; protein: 25 gr; fat: 4 gr.

Ingredients
✓   8 egg whites
✓   30 gr of grated cheddar cheese
✓   2 tbsp of unsweetened almond milk
✓   1 pinch of chilli powder
✓   Salt and pepper to taste
✓   Olive oil

Directions
➢   First, beat egg withes in a bowl.
➢   Add salt, pepper, and chilli powder.
➢   Now, add cheddar cheese too.
➢   Heat the olive oil in a non-stick pan.
➢   When the oil is hot, pour the beaten egg white.
➢   Cook for 3-4 minutes on each side, turning with a plate
➢   Serve the cheddar chili frittata still hot.

Cocoa and soy pancake

Servings: 4 I Prep time: 10 minutes I Cook time: 5 minutes
Nutrition facts per serving: calories: 310; carbs: 8 gr; protein: 14 gr; fat: 6 gr.

Ingredients
✓   60 gr of soy flour
✓   2 eggs
✓   2 tsp of cocoa powder sugar free
✓   4 tbsp of soy yogurt
✓   1 tsp of stevia
✓   1 pinch of baking soda + salt

Directions
➢   Start with the eggs. Separate the yolk from the egg white and transfer them into two different bowls.
➢   Add the stevia to the yolk and beat with a whisk.
➢   Add the soy yogurt and beat again.
➢   Then add the soy flour, baking soda, a pinch of salt and sifted bitter cocoa.
➢   Mix until all the ingredients are smooth.
➢   Then whip the egg whites until stiff and gently incorporate them into the rest of the dough.
➢   Heat a non-stick pan and grease it lightly.
➢   Pour a spoonful of dough for each pancake and wait about a minute.
➢   As soon as the first bubbles form, you can turn them over and continue cooking on the other side.
➢   Serve the pancakes still hot.

Coconut and lime cups

Servings: 4 I Prep time: 15 minutes I Cook time: 5 minutes
Nutrition facts per serving: calories: 320; carbs: 9 gr; protein: 14 gr; fat: 10 gr.

Ingredients
- ✓ 4 eggs
- ✓ 200 gr of coconut flour
- ✓ 1 tbsp of cinnamon
- ✓ 4 tbsp of lime juice + 1 tablespoon of grated lime zest
- ✓ 2 tbsp of melted coconut oil
- ✓ Backing soda + salt

Directions
- ➢ Put the coconut flour in a bowl. Mix with cinnamon, a tsp of baking soda and salt.
- ➢ Combine all the ingredients well.
- ➢ In a separate bowl, beat the eggs until swollen.
- ➢ Add the lime juice, melted coconut oil, beaten eggs and lime zest to the coconut flour mixture.
- ➢ Stir until all the ingredients are well blended.
- ➢ Grease some baking cups with a little coconut oil.
- ➢ Spread the smoothing batter into the bowls.
- ➢ Place in the microwave at high power (800 watts) for about 1 and a half minutes.
- ➢ This is if you decide to cook one cup at a time.
- ➢ If you opt, to save time, cook them all together, cook them for about 3 minutes.
- ➢ Insert a toothpick and if it does not come out dry, bake for another maximum minute until cooked.
- ➢ Serve the cake just warmed for your breakfast.

Coconut light pancake

Servings: 4 I Prep time: 10 minutes I Cook time: 5 minutes
Nutrition facts per serving: calories: 190; carbs:8 gr; protein: 21 gr; fat: 4 gr.

Ingredients
- ✓ 70 gr of coconut flour
- ✓ 4 eggs white
- ✓ 3 drops of liquid stevia
- ✓ 60 ml of sugar-free coconut milk
- ✓ 1 pinch of baking soda + salt

Directions
- ➢ Start placing the eggs white in a large bowl.
- ➢ Add the stevia and beat with a whisk.
- ➢ Add the coconut milk and beat again.
- ➢ Then add the coconut flour and baking soda + a pinch of salt.
- ➢ Mix until all the ingredients are smooth.

- ➢ Heat a non-stick pan and grease it lightly.
- ➢ Pour a spoonful of dough for each pancake and wait about a minute.
- ➢ As soon as the first bubbles form, you can turn them over and continue cooking on the other side.
- ➢ Continue to cook all the pancakes like this.
- ➢ Serve still hot.

Coconut and pistachio pancake

Servings: 4 I Prep time: 15 minutes I Cook time: 5 minutes
Nutrition facts per serving: calories: 220; carbs: 12 gr; protein: 13 gr; fat: 12 gr.

Ingredients
- ✓ 100 gr of coconut flour
- ✓ 4 tbsp of chopped pistachios
- ✓ 2 eggs
- ✓ 2 tsp of stevia
- ✓ 60 ml of unsweetened coconut milk
- ✓ 1 pinch of backing soda + salt

Directions
- ➢ Start dividing the yolk from the egg white and transfer them to two different bowls.
- ➢ Add the stevia to the yolk and beat with a whisk.
- ➢ Also add the coconut milk and continue beating.
- ➢ Then add the coconut flour, a pinch of baking soda + a pinch of salt.
- ➢ Stir until you have a smooth mixture.
- ➢ Then whip the egg whites until stiff and gently incorporate them into the rest of the dough.
- ➢ Heat a non-stick pan and grease it lightly.
- ➢ Pour a spoonful of dough for each pancake and wait about a minute.
- ➢ As soon as the first bubbles form, you can turn them over and continue cooking on the other side.
- ➢ Continue to cook all the pancakes like this.
- ➢ Meanwhile, peel and chop pistachios.
- ➢ Serve pancake turrets chopped pistachios pour over.

Cottage cheese and walnuts truffles

Servings: 4 I Prep time: 10 minutes I Cook time: 25 minutes
Nutrition facts per serving: calories: 130; carbs: 4 gr; protein: 9 gr; fat: 10 gr.

Ingredients
- ✓ 200 gr of cottage cheese
- ✓ 4 tbsp of chopped walnuts

✓ 2 tsp of coconut flour
✓ 1 tsp of extra virgin olive oil
✓ 1 pinch of salt

Directions
➢ First, coarsely chop walnuts, keeping a few whole aside.
➢ Take the cottage cheese from the fridge, put it in a bowl, work it a little with a fork to make it compact.
➢ Add the chopped walnuts and coconut flour, oil, and a pinch of salt.
➢ Mix well, wet your hands, and shape some pralines, arrange them on a tray, decorate them with kernels.
➢ You can serve them directly for breakfast with a coffee.

Cucumber, avocado and soy milk cream

Servings: 4 I Prep time: 15+30 minutes I Cook time: -
Nutrition facts per serving: calories: 250; carbs: 6 gr; protein: 7 gr; fat: 15 gr.

Ingredients
✓ 1 big avocado
✓ 1 big cucumber
✓ 400 of soy milk
✓ 1 tsp of salt
✓ 200 ml of cold broth

Directions
➢ First, halve the avocado, pit it, and remove the pulp from the peel.
➢ Peel and cut the cucumber into slices.
➢ Transfer all the ingredients (avocado, cucumber, lime juice, soy milk, vegetable broth, salt and 1 tbsp of lemon juice) in a measuring container.
➢ Leave to rest in the fridge for about 30 minutes.
➢ After this time, take the ingredients and blend them with an immersion blender.
➢ Blend all ingredients until obtain a thick cream.
➢ Serve your cream for breakfast.

Egg whites and cucumber omelette

Servings: 4 I Prep time: 15 minutes I Cook time: 30 minutes
Nutrition facts per serving: calories: 180; carbs: 4 gr; protein: 25 gr; fat:3 gr.

Ingredients
✓ 8 egg whites
✓ 1 large cucumber
✓ 1 garlic clove

✓ 1 tablespoon of soy milk
✓ 1 pinch of paprika
✓ Olive oil
✓ Salt to taste

Directions
➢ First wash and peel the cucumber.
➢ Cut it in into slices.
➢ Meanwhile, peel and fry the garlic clove in a pan heated with olive oil.
➢ As soon as the garlic has browned, remove it and sauté cucumber slices for about 5 minutes.
➢ While the cucumber slices are cooking, beat the egg whites in a plate and together with the soy milk, pepper, paprika and salt.
➢ Add the cucumber and mix well.
➢ 8. Heat the olive oil in a non-stick pan.
➢ When the oil is hot, pour the beaten egg white with the cucumber.
➢ Cook for 3-4 minutes on each side, turning with a plate.
➢ Serve the cucumber omelette still hot.

Egg and bacon-filled avocado

Servings: 4 I Prep time: 10 minutes I Cook time: 15 minutes
Nutrition facts per serving: calories: 300; carbs: 6 gr; protein: 20 gr; fat: 18 gr.

Ingredients
✓ 4 eggs
✓ 2 avocados
✓ 4 bacon slices
✓ 1 tsp of finely chopped dill
✓ Salt and pepper to taste

Directions
➢ First, preheat the oven to 200°c.
➢ Meanwhile, peel and halve the avocado. Remove the stone and the pulp.
➢ Break the eggs and pour each of them in the middle of the avocado.
➢ Be very careful in this step, you have to make sure that the egg does not come out of the avocado.
➢ Bake in the oven for at least 10/15 minutes.
➢ Check for yourself which egg you like best.
➢ Meanwhile let sauté bacon for 2 minutes in a pan.
➢ When eggs will be ready you can season with salt, pepper and chopped dill.
➢ You can serve your avocado with bacon.

Feta scrambled eggs

Servings: 4 I Prep time: 10 minutes I Cook time: 10 minutes
Nutrition facts per serving: calories: 250; carbs: 1 gr; protein: 21 gr; fat: 4 gr.

Ingredients
- ✓ 6 eggs
- ✓ 60 gr of grated feta cheese
- ✓ 2 tbsp of olive oil
- ✓ Salt and pepper to taste

Directions
- ➤ In a dish, lightly beat the eggs with salt and pepper.
- ➤ Put the eggs in the pan with 1 tbsp of olive oil.
- ➤ Add feta cheese and stir constantly so that the eggs in many separate pieces.
- ➤ Cook for five minutes and then put the eggs in 4 serving dishes.

Serve still hot.

Hazelnut and coconut breakfast cream

Servings: 4 I Prep time: 15 minutes I Cook time: -
Nutrition facts per serving: calories: 280, carbs:10 gr; protein: 16 gr; fat: 8 gr.

Ingredients
- ✓ 400 ml of unsweetened coconut milk
- ✓ 4 tbsp of coconut flour
- ✓ 4 tbsp of chopped hazelnuts
- ✓ 1 pinch of vanilla powder

Directions
- ➤ First, mix the coconut milk, coconut flour, chopped hazelnuts and vanilla in a bowl.
- ➤ Beat the ingredients until the mixture has completely thickened.
- ➤ Pour the mixture equally into 4 bowls.
- ➤ Let it rest for half an hour in the fridge.
- ➤ After this time, take your coconut and hazelnuts creams and serve.

Kale and onion omelette

Servings: 4 I Prep time: 10 minutes I Cook time: 10 minutes
Nutrition facts per serving: calories: 200; carbs:4 gr; protein: 18 gr; fat: 3 gr.
Ingredients
- ✓ 4 eggs
- ✓ 2 tsp of olive oil
- ✓ 1 onion
- ✓ 200 gr of kale
- ✓ Salt and pepper to taste

Directions
- ➤ Start by peeling, washing, and slicing onion.
- ➤ Clean kale too, then cut into pieces.
- ➤ In a small pan, heat the olive oil and sauté the onion for 1 minute, or until aromatic.
- ➤ Stir in the kale and simmer for another 2 minutes, or until it has wilted.
- ➤ Add salt and pepper to taste.
- ➤ Drizzle a little oil into a small non stick frying pan.
- ➤ Season the beaten eggs, then pour them into the pan, stirring and raising the sides to make an omelette that is large and flat.
- ➤ When the bottom of the omelette has browned and the top is almost done, pile the cooked kale onto one side of the omelette and carefully fold over the other half.
- ➤ Slide onto a serving plate and serve your kale omelette.

Maple syrup and cocoa pancake

Servings: 4 I Prep time: 10 minutes I Cook time: 10 minutes
Nutrition facts per serving: calories: 210; carbs:5 gr; protein:12 gr; fat: 14 gr.

Ingredients
- ✓ 60 gr of almond flour
- ✓ 4 tsp sugar free cocoa powder
- ✓ 2 eggs
- ✓ 6 tbsp sugar-free rice milk
- ✓ 4 tsp low-carb sugar free maple syrup
- ✓ Backing soda + salt

Directions
- ➤ Start by placing the egg white into a large bowl.
- ➤ Add the rice milk and beat again.
- ➤ Then add the almond flour, cocoa powder, and a pinch of baking soda + a pinch of salt.
- ➤ Mix until all the ingredients are smooth.
- ➤ Heat a non-stick pan and grease it lightly.
- ➤ Pour a spoonful of dough for each pancake and wait about a minute.
- ➤ After 1 minute, you can turn them over and continue cooking on the other side.
- ➤ Continue to cook all the pancakes like this.
- ➤ Serve the pancakes with a topping off maple syrup.

Mushrooms and parsley omelette

Servings: 4 I Prep time: 10 minutes I Cook time: 10 minutes
Nutrition facts per serving: calories: 250; carbs: 3 gr; protein: 25 gr; fat: 4 gr.

Ingredients
- ✓ 6 eggs
- ✓ 1 tsp of smoked paprika
- ✓ 60 gr of grated parmesan cheese
- ✓ 400 gr of mushrooms
- ✓ 1 tsp of chopped parsley
- ✓ Olive oil
- ✓ Salt and pepper to taste

Directions
- ➤ Start with clearing the mushrooms.
- ➤ Remove the earthy part, wash them, dry them, and cut them into thin slices.
- ➤ Put the eggs in a bowl and beat them vigorously with a fork.
- ➤ Add a pinch of salt, smoked paprika and combine these ingredients very well.
- ➤ In a pan, sauté a drizzle of oil.
- ➤ As soon as it is hot, sauté the mushrooms for 8 minutes.
- ➤ Season with salt and pepper and put them on a plate.
- ➤ Take a non-stick pan.
- ➤ Heat a little oil and then add a little beaten egg.
- ➤ Cook for 2 minutes on each side and then add a little mushroom and the parmesan cheese.
- ➤ Close the omelette, cook for another minute on each side and place it on a serving dish.
- ➤ Repeat the operation until all the eggs are gone.
- ➤ Meanwhile, wash and chop parsley.

Serve hot, sprinkled with chopped parsley.

Oat and coconut pancake

Servings: 4 I Prep time: 15 minutes I Cook time: 30 minutes
Nutrition facts per serving: calories: 170; carbs: 8.9 gr protein: 18 gr; fat: 5 gr.

Ingredients
- ✓ 40 gr of oat flour
- ✓ 2 tbsp of coconut flour
- ✓ 2 eggs white
- ✓ 60 ml of unsweetened coconut milk
- ✓ 1 pinch of baking soda + salt

Directions
- ➤ First, put the egg white into a large bowl, beat with a whisk.
- ➤ Add the coconut milk and beat again.
- ➤ Then add the oat flour, coconut flour, baking soda + a pinch of salt.
- ➤ Mix until all the ingredients are smooth.
- ➤ Heat a non-stick pan and grease it lightly.
- ➤ Pour a spoonful of dough for each pancake and wait about a minute.

- ➤ As soon as the first bubbles form, you can turn them over and continue cooking on the other side.
- ➤ Continue to cook all the pancakes like this.
- ➤ Serve the pancakes still hot.

Oat and courgettes omelette

Servings: 4 I Prep time: 10 minutes I Cook time: 5 minutes
Nutrition facts per serving: calories: 220; carbs: 3 gr; protein: 20 gr; fat: 6 gr.

Ingredients
- ✓ 6 eggs
- ✓ 2 large courgettes
- ✓ 100 gr of oat flakes
- ✓ 4 tbsp of unsweetened oat milk
- ✓ 2 tbsp of grated parmesan cheese
- ✓ Butter
- ✓ Salt to taste

Directions
- ➤ First, wash the courgettes and then cut it into slices.
- ➤ Shell the eggs in a bowl and beat them with a fork.
- ➤ Heat a piece of butter in a pan and cook the courgettes for 10 minutes.
- ➤ Season with salt and pepper and leave to cool.
- ➤ Meanwhile, shell the eggs in a bowl. Add salt, pepper, oat milk, and parmesan. Mix well with the help of a fork.
- ➤ Now add the courgettes and oat flakes and mix everything well.
- ➤ Brush a baking pan with butter and then pour the mixture for the omelette inside.
- ➤ Place the baking pan in the oven and bake at 170° c for 20 minutes.
- ➤ After cooking, remove the pan from the oven and let the omelette rest for 5 minutes.
- ➤ Now cut it into slices, put it on serving plates and serve.

Parmesan and egg white omelette

Servings: 4 I Prep time: 10 minutes I Cook time: 10 minutes
Nutrition facts per serving: calories: 180; carbs: 1 gr; protein: 25 gr; fat:3 gr.

Ingredients
- ✓ 8 egg whites
- ✓ 30 gr of parmesan cheese
- ✓ 2 tbsp of unsweetened oat milk

✓ 1 pinch of nutmeg
✓ Olive oil
✓ Salt and pepper to taste

Directions

➢ First, beat egg withes in a bowl.
➢ Add salt, pepper, and nutmeg.
➢ Finally add parmesan cheese.
➢ Heat the olive oil in a non-stick pan.
➢ When the oil is hot, pour the beaten egg white.
➢ Cook for 3-4 minutes on each side, turning with a plate-like a normal omelette.
➢ Serve the omelette for breakfast still hot.

Porcini and cheddar frittata

Servings: 4 I Prep time: 10 minutes I Cook time: 10 minutes
Nutrition facts per serving: calories: 220; carbs: 4 gr; protein: 21 gr; fat:3 gr.

Ingredients

✓ 4 eggs and 2 egg whites
✓ 1 tsp of chilli powder
✓ 5 tbsp of grated cheddar cheese
✓ 300 gr of porcini mushrooms
✓ Olive oil
✓ Salt and pepper to taste

Directions

➢ First, take porcini mushrooms and remove any earthy part. Then wash porcini, dry them, and cut them into thin slices.
➢ Put the eggs and the egg whites in a bowl and beat them vigorously with a fork.
➢ Add a pinch of salt, chilli powder then mixes the ingredients well.
➢ In a pan, sauté a drizzle of oil.
➢ As soon as it is hot, sauté the porcini mushrooms for 8 minutes.
➢ Season with salt and pepper and put them on a plate.
➢ Take a non-stick pan.
➢ Heat a little oil and then add a little beaten egg.
➢ Cook for 2 minutes on each side and then add a little mushroom and the cheddar cheese.
➢ Close the omelette, cook for another minute on each side and place it on a serving dish.
➢ Repeat the operation until all the eggs are gone.
➢ Serve you porcini frittata still hot.

Scrambled eggs with spinach and ham

Servings: 4 I Prep time: 10 minutes I Cook time: 10 minutes
Nutrition facts per serving: calories: 260; carbs:3 gr, protein: 23 gr fat:12 gr.

Ingredients

✓ 6 eggs
✓ 4 ham slices
✓ 300 gr of spinach leaves
✓ 2 tbsp parmesan grated cheese
✓ Olive oil
✓ Salt and pepper to taste

Directions

➢ First, wash and dry the spinach leaves.
➢ Meanwhile, cut ham slice into little pieces.
➢ Take a non-stick pan and heat the oil.
➢ When it is hot, add the spinach and brown it for 4 minutes, seasoning with salt and pepper.
➢ Add the sliced ham and let cook for other 2 minutes.
➢ In a dish, lightly beat the eggs and after 5 minutes put the eggs in the pan with the spinach and ham.
➢ Add parmesan cheese and stir constantly so that the eggs in many separate pieces.
➢ Cook for five minutes and then put the eggs in serving dishes.
➢ Serve your eggs still hot.

Scrambled eggs with cheddar and courgettes

Servings: 4 I Prep time: 10 minutes I Cook time: 120minutes
Nutrition facts per serving: calories: 320; carbs: 6 gr; protein: 20 gr; fat: 16 gr.

Ingredients

✓ 6 eggs
✓ 2 courgettes
✓ 60 gr of grated cheddar cheese
✓ 1 pinch of smoked paprika
✓ 1 tsp chopped parsley
✓ Olive oil
✓ Salt to taste

Directions

➢ Start by washing and peeling courgettes.
➢ Cut courgettes into little slices.
➢ Take a non-stick pan and heat the oil.
➢ When it is hot, add the courgettes and brown it for 4 minutes, seasoning with salt and smoked paprika.
➢ Add water and let cook for other 10 minutes or until water will be absorbed.
➢ Let courgettes drain.

- In a dish, lightly beat the eggs and after 5 minutes put the eggs in the pan with courgettes and cheddar cheese.
- Stir constantly so that the eggs in many separate pieces.
- Cook for five minutes and then place the eggs into a serving plate.
- Meanwhile, wash and chop parsley.
- Serve hot sprinkled with chopped parsley.

Shallot and bell peppers omelette

Servings: 4 I Prep time: 10 minutes I Cook time: 10 minutes
Nutrition facts per serving: calories: 250; carbs: 10 gr; protein: 13 gr; fat: 7 gr.

Ingredients
- ✓ 4 eggs
- ✓ 2 tbsp of butter
- ✓ 1 shallot
- ✓ 2 red bell peppers
- ✓ Olive oil
- ✓ Salt to taste

Directions
- Start by peeling, washing, and chopping shallot.
- Wash both bell peppers, then remove the cap and seeds.
- Slice bell peppers very thinly.
- In a small saucepan, add the oil and sauté the shallot for 1 minute, or until aromatic.
- Cook for 5 minutes, or until all of the liquid has evaporated, before adding the bell peppers.
- Season with salt.
- Heat a small non-stick frying pan with 1 tbsp of oil.
- Season the beaten eggs, then pour them into the pan, swirling and raising the sides to make an omelette that is large and flat.
- When the bottom of the omelette has browned and the top is almost done, add the bell pepper pieces and carefully fold over the other half.
- Slide onto a plate and serve.

Soy and cocoa porridge

Servings: 4 I Prep time: 15 minutes I Cook time: 30 minutes
Nutrition facts per serving: calories: 200; carbs: 7.6 gr; protein: 15 gr; fat: 5 gr.

Ingredients
- ✓ 50 gr of oat flakes
- ✓ 70 gr of soy flour
- ✓ 1 tbsp of sugar free powder cocoa
- ✓ 240 ml of unsweetened soy milk
- ✓ 40 ml of greek yogurt

Directions
- First, put the oat flakes in a saucepan.
- Add the soy flour, cocoa powder, and combine well all ingredients with a fork.
- Pour in the water and soy milk and mix.
- Turn on the heat and cook until the mixture has thickened, and the flakes are soft.
- Transfer the porridge to a bowl, completing with the soy milk (1 tbsp).
- Serve immediately with 1 tbsp of greek yogurt for porridge.

Soy pancake

Servings: 4 I Prep time: 10 minutes I Cook time: 10 minutes
Nutrition facts per serving: calories: 190; carbs: 9; gr protein:18 gr; fat: 7 gr.

Ingredients
- ✓ 2 eggs white
- ✓ 60 gr of soy flour
- ✓ 60 ml of unsweetened soy milk
- ✓ 1 tbsp of stevia
- ✓ 1 pinch of baking soda + salt

Directions
- First, put the egg white into a large bowl.
- Add the stevia and beat with a whisk.
- Add the soy milk and beat again.
- Then add soy flour and the baking soda + a pinch fo salt.
- Mix until all the ingredients are smooth.
- Heat a non-stick pan and grease it lightly.
- Pour a spoonful of dough for each pancake and wait about a minute.
- As soon as the first bubbles form, you can turn them over and continue cooking on the other side.
- Continue to cook all the pancakes like this.
- Serve the pancakes still hot.

Strawberry oat and pistachio cream

Servings: 4 I Prep time: 10 minutes I Cook time: -
Nutrition facts per serving: calories: 180; carbs: 7.8 gr; protein: 13 gr; fat: 7 gr

Ingredients
- ✓ 400 ml of unsweetened oat milk

- ✓ 4 tbsp of coconut flour
- ✓ 1 cup of strawberries
- ✓ 4 tbsp of chopped pistachio
- ✓ 1 pinch of vanilla powder

Directions
- ➢ First, mix together the oat milk, coconut flour, pistachios and vanilla powder in a bowl.
- ➢ Beat the ingredients until the mixture has completely thickened.
- ➢ Pour the mixture equally into 4 bowls.
- ➢ Let it rest for half an hour in the fridge.
- ➢ In the meantime, wash the strawberries.
- ➢ Serve your cream accompanied by strawberries.

Vanilla and cocoa pancake

Servings: 4 I Prep time: 10 minutes I Cook time: 10 minutes
Nutrition facts per serving: calories: 150; carbs: 5 gr; protein: 11 gr; fat: 10 gr.

Ingredients
- ✓ 60 gr of almond flour
- ✓ 2 eggs
- ✓ 3 tsp of sugar free cocoa powder
- ✓ ½ tbsp sugar-free almond milk
- ✓ ½ tsp vanilla extract

Directions
- ➢ First, separate the yolk from the egg white and transfer them into two different bowls.
- ➢ Add the sweetener drops to the yolk and beat with a whisk.
- ➢ Add the almond milk and beat again.
- ➢ Then add the almond flour, vanilla extract, baking soda and sifted bitter cocoa.
- ➢ Mix until all the ingredients are smooth.
- ➢ Then whip the egg whites until stiff and gently incorporate them into the rest of the dough.
- ➢ Heat a non-stick pan and grease it lightly.
- ➢ Pour a spoonful of dough for each pancake and wait about a minute.
- ➢ After that time, you can turn them over and continue cooking on the other side.
- ➢ Continue to cook all the pancakes like this.
- ➢ Serve the pancakes still hot.

Vanilla soy pancake

Servings: 4 I Prep time: 10 minutes I Cook time: 10 minutes
Nutrition facts per serving: calories: 160; carbs: 3 gr; protein:12 gr; fat: 5 gr.

Ingredients

- ✓ 60 gr of soy flour
- ✓ 2 eggs
- ✓ 1 tsp of stevia
- ✓ 60 ml of unsweetened soy milk
- ✓ 1 tsp of vanilla extract

Directions
- ➢ First, divide the yolk from the egg white and transfer them to two different bowls.
- ➢ Add the stevia to the yolk and beat with a whisk.
- ➢ Add the soy milk too and continue beating.
- ➢ Then add the soy flour, a pinch of baking soda and vanilla extract.
- ➢ Stir until you have a smooth mixture.
- ➢ Then whip the egg whites until stiff and gently incorporate them into the rest of the dough.
- ➢ Heat a non-stick pan and grease it lightly.
- ➢ Pour a spoonful of dough for each pancake and wait about a minute.
- ➢ As soon as the first bubbles form, you can turn them over and continue cooking on the other side.
- ➢ Continue to cook all the pancakes in this way.
- ➢ When your pancakes are well done, serve them.

Starters recipes

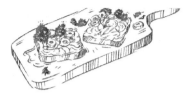

Almond cheddar slices

Servings: 4 I Prep time: 10 minutes I Cook time: 10 minutes
Nutrition facts per serving: calories: 190; carbs: 2 gr; protein: 18 gr; fat: 5 gr.

Ingredients
- ✓ 4 thin slices of cheddar (60 gr about for each)
- ✓ Half an onion
- ✓ 1 clove of garlic
- ✓ 1 cup of vegetable stock
- ✓ 2 tbsp of almond flour
- ✓ Olive oil
- ✓ Salt and pepper to taste

Directions
- ➢ First, peel the onion, wash it, and then cut it into slices.
- ➢ Peel the garlic and then wash it.
- ➢ Put a pan with a little olive oil to heat and then put the garlic to brown.
- ➢ When it is golden brown, remove it and brown the onion slices.
- ➢ Cook the onions for a couple of minutes, stirring constantly.
- ➢ In the meantime, take the cheddar slices and pass them on both sides in the almond flour.
- ➢ Put the slices of cheddar on the onions and cook for two minutes per side.
- ➢ Slowly pour the vegetable broth from the edges and cook over low heat, without ever turning the slices, just make sure they do not stick to the bottom.
- ➢ Season with salt and pepper, turn off and put the slices of cheddar with onions on serving plates.
- ➢ Season with the cooking juices and serve.

Aubergine and grilled provolone

Servings: 4 I Prep time: 10 minutes I Cook time: 10 minutes
Nutrition facts per serving: calories: 295; carbs: 6.7 gr; protein: 22 gr; fat: 6 gr.

Ingredients

- ✓ 120 gr of provolone
- ✓ 1 large aubergine
- ✓ 1 tsp of low-carb soy sauce
- ✓ 10 coriander leaves
- ✓ Olive oil
- ✓ Salt and pepper to taste

Directions
- ➢ First wash and trim the aubergine, then cut them into thin slices and set aside.
- ➢ Take the provolone cheese then cut into slices.
- ➢ Brush the aubergine slices with a little olive oil. Sprinkle with salt and pepper.
- ➢ Heat up a grill and when it is hot, grill the aubergine 3-4 minutes per side.
- ➢ When they are ready put them on a sheet of paper towel and leave them to rest.
- ➢ In the same grill where you cooked the aubergine slices now put the provolone to grill, one minute per side.
- ➢ Wash and dry the coriander leaves.
- ➢ Put them in the glass of the mixer together with a tablespoon of olive oil and the soy sauce.
- ➢ Chop everything very finely.
- ➢ On a serving dish lay the grilled provolone, then on top place 3/4 slices of aubergine.
- ➢ Follow with another layer of provolone and aubergine.
- ➢ Spread the sauce on the surface of the dish and serve.

Avocado salmon and orange skewers

Servings: 4 I Prep time: 20 minutes I Cook time: -
Nutrition facts per serving: calories: 310; carbs: 4 gr; protein: 27 gr; fat: 16 gr.

Ingredients
- ✓ 200 gr of salmon fillet
- ✓ 1 avocado
- ✓ 1 blood orange
- ✓ 1 tbsp of chopped mint leaves
- ✓ Pepper to taste

Directions
- ➢ First, to eliminate any bacteria from the fish, leave the salmon in the freezer for at least two hours.
- ➢ Then take it out, rinse it and dry it.
- ➢ Proceed to cut it into cubes or strips that can be inserted into the skewer.
- ➢ Prepare the sauce for the skewers by pounding mint leaves in a mortar.
- ➢ Put it in a small bowl and mix it with the orange juice and pepper.

➤ Meanwhile wash and peel the avocado, removing central stone.
➤ Cut it into small pieces or cubes.
➤ You can form the skewers with strips (or salmon cubes) alternating it with the avocado ones.
➤ You can serve directly on a serving dish accompanied with the lime and spice sauce.

Avocado almonds and feta salad

Servings: 4 I Prep time: 15 minutes I Cook time: -
Nutrition facts per serving: calories: 270; carbs: 3.7 gr; protein: 23 gr; fat: 9 gr.

Ingredients
✓ 400 gr of feta
✓ 2 avocado
✓ 8 tbsp of chopped almonds
✓ 2 oranges
✓ 10 cherry tomatoes
✓ Olive oil
✓ Salt and pepper to taste

Directions
➤ First, take the feta, and cut it into cubes.
➤ Peel the avocado, wash, and halve it, removing the central stone.
➤ Cut the pulp into cubes and then put it in a bowl.
➤ Season the avocado with the orange juice.
➤ Wash cherry tomatoes and then halve. Put them in the bowl with the avocado.
➤ Add the cubed feta and almonds to the bowl.
➤ Season salt and pepper, a tablespoon of olive oil.
➤ Combine well all ingredients, sprinkle with chopped almonds and serve as starter.

Cottage cheese and basil stuffed courgette

Servings: 4 I Prep time: 20 minutes I Cook time: 10 minutes
Nutrition facts per serving: calories: 220; carbs. 4 gr; protein: 18 gr; fat: 6 gr.

Ingredients
✓ 4 little courgettes
✓ 2 eggs
✓ 200 gr of cottage cheese
✓ 4 tbsp of grated cheddar cheese
✓ 4 basil leaves
✓ Olive oil
✓ Salt to taste

Directions

➤ First, peel the courgettes, wash, and dry them.
➤ Then cut them in half lengthwise.
➤ Remove the internal pulp with a spoon without damaging the external part.
➤ Set the inside pulp aside.
➤ Wash and chop basil leaves.
➤ Put the cottage cheese, the eggs, a bit of almond flour, chopped basil, 1 tbsp of cheddar cheese and the internal pulp of the courgette in a bowl.
➤ Mix the ingredients to obtain a homogeneous and velvety mixture.
➤ Season with salt and pepper and mix again.
➤ Fill the courgette with the mixture and then place them in a pan brushed with a little olive oil.
➤ Let cook in the preheated oven at 200°c for 10 minutes.
➤ As soon as they are cooked, take them out of the oven, put them on serving plates and serve as a starter.

Cucumber flax seeds and rocket salad

Servings: 4 I Prep time: 10 minutes I Cook time: -
Nutrition facts per serving: calories: 90; carbs: 6 gr; protein:3 gr; fat: 3 gr.

Ingredients
✓ 160 gr of rocket salad
✓ 1 cucumber
✓ 1 tsp of flax seeds
✓ 2 tsp of apple cider vinegar
✓ 1 tsp of olive oil
✓ Salt to taste

Directions
➤ First, clean and wash the rocket salad.
➤ Meanwhile wash and peel cucumber.
➤ Then cut the cucumber into slices.
➤ Combine the cucumber slices, the rocket salad and flax seeds in a bowl or serving dish.
➤ Season with the oil, salt and vinegar and mix well before serving.

Endive, cheese, and soy flan

Servings: 4 I Prep time: 15 minutes I Cook time: 60 minutes
Nutrition facts per serving: calories: 200; carbs: 2 gr; protein: 15 gr fat: 8 gr.

Ingredients
✓ 600 gr of endive
✓ 250 ml of soy milk
✓ 2 tbsp of soy flour

✓ 2 tbsp of grated parmesan cheese
✓ 100 gr of cream cheese

Directions
➢ First, wash the endive well and then let it blanch by putting it in boiling salted water for a few minutes.
➢ Drain and cut into small pieces.
➢ Meanwhile, peel a piece of shallot and chop it.
➢ Put it now on the fire in a saucepan with olive oil, add piece of shallot.
➢ Season by wetting every now and then with soy milk and cook until it is almost undone
➢ Remove it from the heat and pass it to the mill to dry it.
➢ Now add two tablespoons of soy flour dissolved in two tablespoons of water, the grated parmesan cheese and finally the cream cheese.
➢ Season with salt and pepper and pour the mixture into a greased and lightly floured mould. Cook in a bain-marie for about 40 minutes.
➢ Serve the flan still hot as starter.

Green beans pistachio and feta salad

Servings: 4 I Prep time: 15 minutes I Cook time: -
Nutrition facts per serving: calories: 270, carbs: 4 gr; protein: 26 gr; fat: 10 gr.

Ingredients
✓ 1 cup of green beans
✓ 100 gr of feta
✓ Half a red onion
✓ 4 tbsp of chopped pistachios
✓ Olive oil, salt and pepper to taste

Directions
➢ First, remove the tips from the green beans and then wash them.
➢ Bring a pot of water and salt to a boil and then cook the beans for 10 minutes.
➢ Peel the half red onion wash it and cut it into slices.
➢ Cut the feta into pieces.
➢ Take a grill and when it is hot, grill the feta for 2 minutes per side.
➢ Put the feta on a cutting board and cut it into cubes.
➢ Drain the green beans and put them in a bowl.
➢ Add the red onion and season with oil, salt, and pepper.
➢ Mix and then transfer the vegetables to serving dishes.
➢ Sprinkle with feta and pistachios and serve.

Nuts and cheese truffles

Servings: 4 I Prep time: 10 minutes I Cook time: 10 minutes
Nutrition facts per serving: calories: 315; carbs: 6 gr; protein: 21 gr; fat: 18 gr.

Ingredients
✓ 300 gr of cream cheese
✓ 2 tbsp of chopped pecans
✓ 1 tbsp of chopped hazelnuts
✓ 1 pinch of spicy paprika
✓ Olive oil
✓ Pinch of salt

Directions
➢ Start by taking creamy cheese and transfer it into a food processor.
➢ Before blending, season it with oil, and a pinch of paprika and salt, and blend until a smooth and homogeneous cream is obtained.
➢ In a bowl, mix the cheese cream with pecans and hazelnuts, kneading until a workable mixture is obtained, then take a little dough at a time and form small balls slightly larger than a walnut, which you will arrange on a plate.
➢ On a cutting board, chop other pecans and hazelnuts with a sharp knife.
➢ Combine both in a plate.
➢ Then pass each truffle in this nuts mixture so as to completely cover the surface.
➢ Now, you can serve your truffles as starters.

Peanuts and tofu pralines

Servings: 4 I Prep time: 10 minutes I Cook time: -
Nutrition facts per serving: calories: 200; carbs: 5 gr; protein: 19 gr; fat: 4 gr.

Ingredients
✓ 400 gr of tofu
✓ 4 tbsp of chopped peanuts
✓ 2 tsp of olive oil
✓ 1 pinch of paprika
✓ Salt, a pinch

Directions
➢ First, coarsely chop the peanuts, keeping a few whole aside.
➢ Take the tofu cheese, put it in a bowl, work it a little with a fork to make it compact.
➢ Add the chopped peanuts, a pinch of paprika, oil, and salt.
➢ Mix well, wet your hands, and shape the pralines, arrange them on a tray.
➢ You can serve them directly as starter.

Rocket salmon and fennel seeds salad

Servings: 4 I Prep time: 10 minutes I Cook time: -
Nutrition facts per serving: calories: 210; carbs: 2 gr; protein: 26 gr; fat: 4 gr.

Ingredients
- ✓ 8 slices of smoked salmon
- ✓ 200 gr of rocket salad
- ✓ 2 tbsp of apple cider vinegar
- ✓ 1 tbsp of fennel seeds
- ✓ Olive oil
- ✓ Salt and pepper to taste

Directions
- ➢ First, cut smoked salmon into pieces.
- ➢ Meanwhile, wash and dry the rocket salad.
- ➢ Take a salad bowl and put salmon strips and rocket salad.
- ➢ Add a pinch of salt and pepper and mix.
- ➢ Season the salad with olive oil and apple cider vinegar, season with salt and pepper, sprinkle with fennel seeds and serve your starter.

Tofu and pineapple starter

Servings: 4 I Prep time: 10 minutes I Cook time: 20 minutes
Nutrition facts per serving: calories: 160; carbs:9 gr; protein:16 gr; fat: 2 gr.

Ingredients
- ✓ 250 gr of tofu
- ✓ 1 lime
- ✓ 4 tbsp of pineapple juice
- ✓ Olive oil
- ✓ Salt and pepper to taste

Directions
- ➢ Rinse and pat the tofu with a kitchen paper, then cut it into slices.
- ➢ Put a little olive oil in a pan and as soon as it is hot, cook the slices of tofu, two minutes per side.
- ➢ Put the slices aside and in the same pan put the filtered lime and pineapple juice.
- ➢ Bring to a boil, season with salt and pepper and mix.
- ➢ Now put the slices of tofu in the pan, let them flavour for a couple of minutes and then turn off.
- ➢ Put the slices on serving plates, sprinkle with the cooking juices and serve your starter.

Tomato olive and cottage cheese salad

Servings: 4 I Prep time: 10 minutes I Cook time: -
Nutrition facts per serving: calories: 290; carbs: 5.8 gr; protein: 28 gr; fat: 9 gr.

Ingredients
- ✓ 200 gr of cottage cheese
- ✓ 12 green olives
- ✓ 10 cherry tomatoes
- ✓ Olive oil to taste
- ✓ 2 tbsp of apple cider vinegar
- ✓ Salt to taste

Directions
- ➢ First, rinse the cottage cheese.
- ➢ Cut the cottage cheese into pieces.
- ➢ Now, wash cherry tomatoes then halve.
- ➢ Take two bowls and put the slices of cottage cheese in the centre, then the halved cherry tomatoes and finally the pitted green olives.
- ➢ Season everything with oil, salt, and apple cider vinegar.
- ➢ Sprinkle with a bit of chopped basil grains and serve.

Tuna and feta radicchio salad

Servings: 4 I Prep time: 10 minutes I Cook time: -
Nutrition facts per serving: calories: 320; carbs: 3 gr; protein: 29 gr; fat: 8 gr.

Ingredients
- ✓ 200 gr of tuna in oil
- ✓ 120 gr of feta
- ✓ 200 gr of radicchio leaves
- ✓ Olive oil to taste
- ✓ Salt and pepper to taste

Directions
- ➢ First, drain tuna e cut into pieces with a fork.
- ➢ Cut the feta into cubes.
- ➢ Wash and dry the radicchio well and then cut it into small pieces.
- ➢ Put the radicchio leaves in a bowl and season with oil, salt, and pepper.
- ➢ Now divide the radicchio into 4 serving plates.
- ➢ Place the piece of tuna and feta on top.
- ➢ Drizzle with a drizzle of oil and serve.

Turkey tomatoes and lettuce salad

Servings: 4 I Prep time: 10 minutes I Cook time: -

Nutrition facts per serving: calories: 280; carbs: 8.8 gr; protein: 26 gr; fat: 4 gr.

Ingredients
- ✓ 12 slices of turkey roast
- ✓ A bunch of lettuce
- ✓ 12 cherry tomatoes
- ✓ 2 tbsp of apple cider vinegar
- ✓ 1 sprig of thyme
- ✓ Olive oil
- ✓ Salt and pepper to taste

Directions
- ➢ First, wash and thyme.
- ➢ Take the roasted turkey and cut into pieces.
- ➢ Meanwhile, wash and dry the lettuce and then cut it into thin strips.
- ➢ Wash and dry the cherry tomatoes and cut them in half.
- ➢ Take a salad bowl and put a pinch of salt and pepper inside the vegetables and mix.
- ➢ Put the roasted turkey in the salad bowl together with the vegetables.
- ➢ Season the salad with olive oil and apple cider vinegar, season with salt and pepper if necessary and then serve as starter.

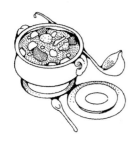

Main courses recipes

Meat dishes

Poultry recipes

***

Almond and feta turkey

Servings: 4 I Prep time: 10 minutes I Cook time: 15 minutes
Nutrition facts per serving: calories: 380; carbs: 5 gr; protein: 38 gr; fat: 13 gr.

Ingredients:
- ✓ 4 slices of turkey breast (200 gr for each)
- ✓ 2 tbsp of chopped almonds
- ✓ 2 tbsp of grated feta cheese
- ✓ 1 tsp of fresh coriander
- ✓ 1 tbsp of olive oil
- ✓ Salt and pepper to taste

Directions
- ➤ First, start with cleaning the turkey breast.
- ➤ Remove the excess fat and then if the slices are not thin enough, thin them with a meat mallet.
- ➤ Wash and dry the slices with kitchen paper towel and then sprinkle them on both sides with salt and pepper.
- ➤ Wash and dry the coriander.
- ➤ Peel and finely chop almonds.
- ➤ Mix the chopped almonds with the feta cheddar cheese and coriander.
- ➤ Pass the slices over the breading, pressing them to make the breading adhere well.
- ➤ Heat the olive oil in a pan and as soon as it is hot, put the turkey to brown.
- ➤ Turn them over and cook until the meat is well cooked and golden on the outside.
- ➤ Serve the crusted turkey immediately and hot, sprinkled with the cooking juices.

Asparagus turkey

Servings: 4 I Prep time: 10 minutes I Cook time: 20 minutes
Nutrition facts per serving: calories: 245; carbs: 2 gr; protein: 29 gr; fat: 3 gr.

Ingredients
- ✓ 600 gr of sliced turkey breast
- ✓ 300 gr of asparagus
- ✓ 2 tbsp of almond flour
- ✓ Olive oil, salt and pepper to taste

Directions
- ➤ Start with the asparagus. Wash them under running water and remove the hard underside.
- ➤ Take a saucepan and boil 500 ml of salted water.
- ➤ When it comes to a boil, put the asparagus, and cook for about ten minutes, adjusting with salt and pepper. They should not be overcooked; they should remain crunchy.
- ➤ Wash and dry the turkey slices and then pass them over the almond flour.
- ➤ Heat a little olive oil in a pan and as soon as it is hot enough, brown the slices of meat.
- ➤ Turn them a couple of times. Season with salt and pepper and as soon as they are cooked, remove them from the heat and keep them warm.
- ➤ Take two serving plates and put the asparagus on the bottom. Season with a drizzle of olive oil and arrange the slices of turkey on top.

Avocado turkey

Servings: 4 I Prep time: 10 minutes I Cook time: 15 minutes marinated + 15 minutes cooking
Nutrition facts per serving: calories: 360; carbs: 8 gr; protein: 38 gr; fat: 12 gr.

Ingredients
- ✓ 500 gr of turkey slices
- ✓ ½ orange
- ✓ 1 avocado
- ✓ 1 pinch of smoked paprika
- ✓ Olive oil, salt and pepper

Directions
- ➤ First, wash and dry the turkey slices.
- ➤ Put the turkey to a fairly large pan and season with oil, salt pepper and paprika.
- ➤ Strain the juice from the orange, then sprinkle the turkey slices.
- ➤ Cover with transparent paper and put them in the fridge for 15 minutes to marinate.
- ➤ Peel the half avocado, remove the stone, wash it, dry it and then cut it into cubes. Season with oil, salt and pepper.
- ➤ After 15 minutes, remove the turkey from the fridge.

➢ Heat a grill, which should be hot, and cook the slices for 3 minutes per side. The turkey should be well cooked and have grill streaks on the surface.

➢ Transfer the turkey to a serving plate and garnish with the flavour avocado.

Avocado and rocket lime chicken salad

Servings: 4 I Prep time: 20 minutes I Cook time: 15 minutes
Nutrition facts per serving: calories: 480; carbs: 5 gr; protein: 46 gr; fat: 13 gr.

Ingredients
➢ 1 chicken breast (600 gr about)
➢ 200 gr of rocket salad
➢ 1 avocado
➢ 1 lime
➢ Olive oil, salt and pepper to taste

Directions
✓ First, wash and dry the chicken and remove excess fat.
✓ Brush the meat with olive oil and season with salt and pepper.
✓ Heat a plate and when it is hot, put the chicken to grill.
✓ Cook for 6 minutes around on each side and then remove the meat from the grill.
✓ Put the chicken on a plate and leave it aside to cool.
✓ Meanwhile, wash and dry the rocket salad.
✓ Peel the avocado, remove the stone, and then cut the pulp into slices.
✓ Now cut the chicken breast into thin strips.
✓ Put the rocket salad on the bottom of the serving dish.
✓ Add the avocado and the chicken.
✓ In a bowl, mix the filtered lime juice, salt, oil, and pepper.
✓ Sprinkle the salad with the emulsion and serve it.

Cheese sauce almond turkey

Servings: 4 I Prep time: 10 minutes I Cook time: 20 minutes
Nutrition facts per serving: calories 395; carbs: 1.5 gr; protein: 40 gr; fat: 7 gr.

Ingredients
✓ 800 gr of sliced turkey breast
✓ 100 gr of cheddar cheese
✓ 50 ml of no sugar almond milk
✓ 2 tbsp of almond flour
✓ Salt and pepper to taste

Directions
➢ Start by cutting the cheddar into cubes and putting it in a bowl with the almond milk.
➢ Set the bowl aside and let it rest for an hour.
➢ Wash and dry the turkey slices and then pass them over the almond flour.
➢ Heat a little olive oil in a pan and as soon as it is hot enough, brown the slices of meat.
➢ Turn them a couple of times. Season with salt and pepper and as soon as they are cooked, remove them from the heat and keep them warm.
➢ After the resting time, put the cheddar and milk in a saucepan. Melt the cheddar over low heat and as soon as you have a thick and homogeneous sauce turn off the heat.
➢ Take two serving plates place oat turkey slices. Then sprinkle everything with the cheese sauce and serve.

Chicken and veggies

Servings: 4 I Prep time: 10 minutes I Cook time: 20 minutes
Nutrition facts per serving: calories: 480; carbs: 5 gr; protein: 42 gr; fat: 7 gr.

Ingredients
✓ 600 gr of chicken breast
✓ 300 gr of broccoli florets
✓ 150 gr of spinach
✓ 100 gr of shredded cheddar cheese
✓ 2 garlic cloves
✓ Olive oil
✓ Salt to taste

Directions
➢ Start the recipe by wash and dry the chicken breast, then cut it into slices.
➢ Meanwhile, wash broccoli taking only florets.
➢ Wash spinach leaves too.
➢ Peel and mince garlic cloves.
➢ In a large saucepan, heat 1 tablespoon olive oil over medium-high heat.
➢ Cook for 4-5 minutes, or until the chicken is golden and well cooked inside. Sauté for another minute, or until the garlic is fragrant.
➢ Add broccoli florets, spinach leaves and shredded cheddar cheese.
➢ Cook for another 5 minutes until the broccoli is well cooked.
➢ Serve you chicken dish still hot.

Chicken with bell peppers

Servings: 4 I Prep time: 15 minutes I Cook time: 10 minutes
Nutrition facts per serving: calories: 360; carbs: 9 gr; protein: 32 gr; fat: 2 gr.

Ingredients
- ✓ 700 gr of chicken breast
- ✓ ½ shallot
- ✓ 2 red bell peppers
- ✓ 20 ml of apple cider vinegar
- ✓ Olive oil
- ✓ Salt and pepper to taste

Directions
- ➢ Start by washing, removing seeds, and slicing both bell peppers.
- ➢ Wash and chop shallot.
- ➢ Now, season the chicken.
- ➢ To prevent overcrowding the skillet, which will inhibit browning, split the chicken in half and cook it in two batches.
- ➢ In a skillet, sear half of it in the oil.
- ➢ Reduce the heat under the skillet and repeat with the remaining chicken, adding additional oil as needed.
- ➢ Remove the chicken from the skillet and place both batches on a platter covered with foil.
- ➢ Now, sauté the peppers and shallot in a pan.
- ➢ Add both to the skillet and cook them.
- ➢ Cook, stirring frequently, until they're soft and beginning to brown. They'll become fragrant within about one minute.
- ➢ Add in the vinegar, and let it evaporate.
- ➢ Finish cooking the chicken in the sauce
- ➢ Now add the chicken back into the skillet with any accumulated juices from the plate and bring it all up to a simmer.
- ➢ Then just simmer on medium-low heat to thicken the sauce and cook the chicken all the way through.
- ➢ Serve your chicken with bell peppers still hot.

Green bean and roasted chicken salad

Servings: 4 I Prep time: 10 minutes I Cook time: 10 minutes
Nutrition facts per serving: calories: 270; carbs: 6 gr; protein: 30 gr; fat:12 gr.

Ingredients
- ✓ 250 gr of green beans
- ✓ 16 slices of roasted chicken
- ✓ 8 leaves of radicchio
- ✓ 2 tsp of mustard
- ✓ 2 tsp of apple cider vinegar
- ✓ Olive oil, salt and pepper

Directions
- ➢ Remove the tips from the green beans, then wash them and let them drain.
- ➢ Bring a pot of water and salt to a boil and then boil the green beans for 10 minutes.
- ➢ Once cooked, drain, and let them cool.
- ➢ Meanwhile, wash and dry the radicchio and then cut them into small pieces.
- ➢ Place the chicken on a cutting board and cut it into thin slices.
- ➢ Put the chicken, green beans, radicchio in a salad bowl.
- ➢ In a small bowl, emulsify the mustard, oil, salt, pepper, and apple cider vinegar.
- ➢ Sprinkle the salad with the emulsion, combine well and serve.

Leek and pistachio turkey

Servings: 4 I Prep time: 20 minutes I Cook time: 20 minutes
Nutrition facts per serving: calories: 340; carbs: 5 gr; protein: 41; gr fat: 11 gr.

Ingredients
- ✓ 800 gr of turkey breast
- ✓ 4 tbsp of chopped pistachios
- ✓ 2 tbsp of apple cider vinegar
- ✓ 1 leek
- ✓ 1 clove of garlic
- ✓ Olive oil, salt and pepper to taste

Directions
- ➢ First, rinse the leek under running water and remove the outer leaves.
- ➢ Cut the end that has the root and the other end with the dark green leaves, and then slice it thinly.
- ➢ Wash and dry the turkey, remove the excess fat, and then cut it into cubes.
- ➢ Peel and wash the garlic and then chop it.
- ➢ Put the pistachios in a non-stick pan and toast them for a couple of minutes.
- ➢ Heat a tbsp of olive oil in another pan.
- ➢ When it is hot, put the garlic to brown.
- ➢ Add the turkey cubes and mix.
- ➢ Sauté the turkey for a couple of minutes and then add the leek and vinegar.
- ➢ Stir, sauté 2 minutes and then add half a glass of water.
- ➢ Continue cooking for another 10 minutes.
- ➢ Season with salt and pepper, add the chopped pistachios.
- ➢ Combine well ingredients and then turn off.

➤ Put the pistachio turkey on serving plates, sprinkle with the cooking juices and serve.

Mushroom yogurt sauce chicken

Servings: 4 I Prep time: 15 minutes I Cook time: 25 minutes
Nutrition facts per serving: calories: 295; carbs: 5 gr; protein: 30 gr; fat: 6 gr.

Ingredients
✓ 600 gr of chicken breast
✓ 250 gr of mushrooms
✓ 120 ml of greek yogurt
✓ 1 garlic clove
✓ 1 pinch of smoked paprika
✓ Olive oil, salt and pepper to taste

Directions
➤ First, peel and wash the garlic.
➤ Remove the earthy part of the mushrooms, wash them under running water, dry them and then cut them into slices.
➤ Clean the chicken breast, remove excess fat and then cut into two slices. Wash it and dry it.
➤ Heat the olive oil in a pan. As soon as it is hot, brown the garlic and then remove it.
➤ Place the chicken slices and brown them on both sides until they are well cooked. Season with salt and pepper and paprika.
➤ Remove the chicken and keep it warm.
➤ Now add the mushrooms to the pan where you cooked the chicken.
➤ Brown them for 10 minutes and then add the greek yogurt. Stir to mix well.
➤ Let the sauce reduce and then season with salt and pepper. Add the chicken fillet, let it flavour and then turn off the heat.
➤ Serve the fillet sprinkled with the mushroom sauce.

Olives and mushrooms turkey

Servings: 4 I Prep time: 15 minutes I Cook time: 20 minutes
Nutrition facts per serving: calories: 420; carbs: 5 gr, protein: 44 gr; fat: 11 gr.

Ingredients
✓ 800 gr of turkey breast
✓ 400 gr of mushrooms
✓ 12 pitted black olives
✓ 3 tbsp of vegetable broth
✓ 1 garlic clove
✓ Olive oil, salt and pepper to taste

Directions
➤ Start with cleaning the mushrooms. Remove the earthy part, rinse them quickly under running water and then dry them. Cut them into thin slices.
➤ Peel and wash the garlic.
➤ Switch to the turkey. Remove any residues of skin, fat and bones and then cut it into many thin strips.
➤ Put the olive oil in a pan and as soon as it is hot, add the garlic. Fry it until completely pierced and then add the mushrooms.
➤ Cook the mushrooms over medium heat for 10 minutes, seasoning with salt and pepper, then remove the garlic and add the turkey.
➤ Cook for another 8 minutes, adding a little turkey broth from time to time.
➤ After 8 minutes, add the olives and cook for another two minutes, seasoning with salt and pepper.
➤ Remove the turkey from the pan and place it with the mushrooms and olives on two serving plates.
➤ Stir in the cooking juices of the turkey, reduce it, and then sprinkle the turkey with the sauce.

Orange and rosemary chicken

Servings: 4 I Prep time: 15 minutes I Cook time: 20 minutes
Nutrition facts per serving: calories: 340; carbs: 5 gr; protein: 34 gr; fat: 2 gr.

Ingredients
✓ 4 slices of chicken breast (150 gr for each)
✓ 1 orange
✓ 2 sprigs of rosemary
✓ 2 tbsp of apple cider vinegar
✓ Olive oil, salt and pepper to taste

Directions
➤ First, beat the chicken slices with a meat mallet. This operation is to make them thinner and more homogeneous.
➤ After that wash them under running water and let dry.
➤ Brush a pan with olive oil and put the chicken slices inside, season with salt and pepper.
➤ Squeeze the orange and then cover the chicken with the filtered orange juice.
➤ Wash and dry the thyme and then take the needles and place them on the chicken.
➤ Finish sprinkles the meat with apple cider vinegar and cook in the oven at 210°c for 15 minutes.
➤ When chicken is done, remove the pan from the oven and let the meat rest for a couple of minutes.

➢ Put the meat on serving plates, sprinkle it with the cooking juices and serve.

Pistachio and parmesan chicken

Servings: 4 I Prep time: 15 minutes I Cook time: 15 minutes
Nutrition facts per serving: calories:410; carbs: 7 gr; protein: 40 gr; fat: 8 gr.

Ingredients
✓ 4 slices of chicken breast (150 gr for each)
✓ 60 of chopped pistachios
✓ 60 gr of grated parmesan cheese
✓ 1 tbsp of olive oil
✓ Salt and pepper to taste

Directions
➢ First, start with the chicken breast.
➢ Remove the excess fat and then if the slices are not thin enough, thin them with a meat mallet.
➢ Wash and dry the slices with kitchen paper towel and then sprinkle them on both sides with salt and pepper.
➢ Peel and finely chop pistachios.
➢ Mix together the chopped pistachios with the grated parmesan cheese.
➢ Pass the slices over the pistachio and parmesan flour, pressing them to make the breading adhere well.
➢ Heat the olive oil in a pan and as soon as it is hot, put the chicken to brown.
➢ Turn them over and cook until the meat is well cooked and golden on the outside.
➢ Serve the crusted chicken immediately and hot, sprinkled with the cooking juices.

Spicy turkey

Servings: 4 I Prep time: 10 minutes I Cook time: 40 minutes
Nutrition facts per serving: calories: 220; carbs:1 gr; protein: 30 gr; fat: 1 gr.

Ingredients
✓ 800 gr of turkey breast
✓ 2 tbsp of mixed spices
✓ 2 tbsp of grated ginger (or powdered ginger)
✓ Olive oil
✓ Salt to taste

Directions
➢ First clean the turkey breast, removing any bones or fat excess.
➢ Rub the turkey with the olive oil and season them with the spices and ginger.

➢ Rub half tablespoon of oil over the skin side of the turkey after seasoning both sides.
➢ Preheat the oven at 190ºC.
➢ Put turkey breast in the baking pan and place in the oven.
➢ Place the pan in the oven and let cook for 30 minutes.
➢ Turn every 10 minutes.
➢ Let it rest 10 minutes before carving.
➢ Serve turkey still hot.

Thyme chicken and lettuce salad

Servings: 4 I Prep time: 15 minutes I Cook time: 30 minutes
Nutrition facts per serving: calories: 320; carbs: 5 gr; protein: 32 gr; fat: 2 gr.

Ingredients
✓ 600 gr of chicken breast
✓ 200 gr of lettuce
✓ 12 cherry tomatoes
✓ 3 tbsp of apple cider vinegar
✓ 1 sprig of thyme
✓ Olive oil
✓ Salt and pepper to taste

Directions
➢ First, wash and dry thyme.
➢ Take the chicken breast, remove any fat, skin and bones, and then wash it under running water. Dry it and halve.
➢ Take a pot, put 200 ml of water, add salt, and bring it to a boil. Place a steamer basket or alternatively a large colander on the pot.
➢ Place the chicken, sage and rosemary in the basket. Cook for 25 minutes, seasoning with salt and pepper.
➢ After the Cook time, turn off and let the meat cool.
➢ Meanwhile, wash and dry the lettuce and then cut it into thin strips.
➢ Wash and dry the cherry tomatoes and halve them.
➢ Take a salad bowl and put a pinch of salt and pepper inside the vegetables and mix.
➢ Take the chicken, which has cooled in the meantime, and cut it into cubes.
➢ Put it in the salad bowl together with the vegetables.
➢ Season the salad with olive oil and apple cider vinegar, salt, and pepper.
➢ Serve your chicken salad.

Beef and veal recipes

***

Asparagus baked beef

Servings: 4 I Prep time: 15 minutes I Cook time: 20 minutes
Nutrition facts per serving: calories: 360; carbs: 3 gr; protein: 41 gr; fat: 6 gr.

Ingredients
- ✓ 4 lean beef fillet (150 gr for each)
- ✓ 400 gr of asparagus
- ✓ 1 tsp garlic powder
- ✓ ½ tsp smoked paprika
- ✓ Olive oil
- ✓ Salt and pepper to taste

Directions
- ➤ First, clean the asparagus well.
- ➤ Remove the white part of the stem and keep the more tender tips aside.
- ➤ Now you can take the beef fillet and rinse it under running water.
- ➤ Dry it well with a paper towel.
- ➤ Wash and dry beef fillet too.
- ➤ Season beef fillet with salt and pepper.
- ➤ Season further with garlic powder and smoked paprika.
- ➤ Lightly oil a baking pan and place the asparagus first and then the beef fillet.
- ➤ Bake in a preheated oven at 190° c for about 15/20 minutes.
- ➤ Check both the doneness of both meat and asparagus.
- ➤ When all it's done, serve the beef fillet still warm with the asparagus.

Avocado and orange beef

Servings: 4 I Prep time: 10 minutes I Cook time: 10 minutes
Nutrition facts per serving: calories: 430; carbs: 4 gr; protein: 38 gr; fat: 9 gr.

Ingredients
- ✓ 4 beef fillet (150 gr for each)
- ✓ 1 orange
- ✓ 1 avocado
- ✓ ½ shallot
- ✓ ½ tsp of smoked paprika
- ✓ Olive oil, salt and pepper

Directions
- ➤ First, peel the avocado, remove the central stone, and then wash and dry it.
- ➤ Cut it into cubes.
- ➤ Peel and wash the shallot. Dry it and then chop it.
- ➤ Wash and dry the beef fillet and then cut it into small pieces.
- ➤ Wash and dry the orange, grate the peel, and set it aside and then squeeze the pulp and strain the juice into a bowl.
- ➤ Put the meat, salt, pepper, olive oil, paprika in the bowl with the orange juice.
- ➤ Stir gently to mix everything.
- ➤ Let sauté the beef filet with the sauce for few minutes in a pan.
- ➤ When it will be done, serve the meat in the centre of the dish.
- ➤ Add the avocado cubes and serve.

Beef lime carpaccio with mustard and mushrooms

Servings: 4 I Prep time: 10 minutes + 60 minutes in the fridge of marinating I Cook time: -
Nutrition facts per serving: calories: 160; carbs: 2 gr; protein: 19 gr; fat: 5 gr.

Ingredients
- ✓ 200 gr of very thinly sliced beef
- ✓ 3 tbsp of mustard
- ✓ 200 gr of mushrooms
- ✓ 1 lime, juiced
- ✓ Olive oil, salt and pepper to taste

Directions
- ➤ Start by removing any earthy part of the mushrooms. Wash and dry them and then chop them coarsely.
- ➤ Put the chopped mushrooms in a bowl.
- ➤ Add the mustard, the filtered lime juice, oil, salt, and pepper.
- ➤ Stir until you get a homogeneous mixture.
- ➤ Put the meat in 4 serving plates and season with oil, salt, and pepper.
- ➤ Sprinkle the meat with the sauce and then transfer the dishes to rest in the fridge for 60 minutes.
- ➤ After 60 minutes, remove the lime beef carpaccio from the fridge and serve.

Bell pepper sauce beef

Servings: 4 I Prep time: 10 minutes I Cook time: 90 minutes
Nutrition facts per serving: calories: 460; carbs: 11 gr; protein: 40 gr; fat: 7 gr.

Ingredients
- ✓ 600 gr of beef fillet
- ✓ 1 red pepper
- ✓ 1 yellow pepper
- ✓ 4 basil leaves
- ✓ 5 tbsp of apple cider vinegar
- ✓ Olive oil, salt and pepper to taste

Directions
- ➢ First, wash and dry the beef fillet and then remove all excess fat.
- ➢ Wash and dry the 2 bell peppers.
- ➢ Brush a baking pan and put the peppers inside.
- ➢ Bake in the oven for 30 minutes at 180 °c.
- ➢ Meanwhile, brush another baking pan with olive oil.
- ➢ Brush the loin with olive oil and season with salt and pepper.
- ➢ Put the meat inside the baking pan and, when the peppers have finished cooking, put it in the oven.
- ➢ Raise the oven temperature to 160°c and cook the meat for 60 minutes.
- ➢ Put the peppers to cool, then remove the cap, seeds, and white filaments.
- ➢ Peel them and then cut them into slices.
- ➢ Put the peppers in the blender glass.
- ➢ Wash and dry the basil leaves.
- ➢ Put the basil leaves, 4 tablespoons of olive oil, salt, pepper and 5 tablespoons of apple cider vinegar in the blender along with the peppers.
- ➢ Operate the blender and blend until you get a thick and homogeneous sauce.
- ➢ Once the roast is cooked, remove the baking pan from the oven and let the meat rest for 5 minutes.
- ➢ Put the meat on a cutting board and cut it into thin slices.
- ➢ Put the meat on serving plates, sprinkle it with the bell pepper sauce and serve.

Broccoli and lime beef

Servings: 4 I Prep time: 10 minutes I Cook time: 20 minutes
Nutrition facts per serving: calories: 420; carbs: 4 gr; protein: 42 gr; fat: 7 gr.

Ingredients
- ✓ 600 gr of lean beef fillet
- ✓ 20 broccoli tops
- ✓ 1 sprig of thyme
- ✓ 1 lime juice
- ✓ Olive oil, salt and pepper

Directions
- ➢ First, wash and dry broccoli tops, then cut them into many pieces.
- ➢ Remove any excess fat from the beef, then wash and dry it.
- ➢ Wash and dry thyme sprigs.
- ➢ Wash and strain lime juice.
- ➢ Put the olive oil, lime juice, salt and pepper in a bowl and mix with a fork until you get a homogeneous emulsion.
- ➢ Take one sheet of aluminium foil and place the beef. Add the broccoli, thyme and then wet everything with the oil and lemon emulsion.
- ➢ Close the foil making sure to seal it well.
- ➢ Put in the oven and cook at 180°c for 15/20 minutes.
- ➢ When it is ready, remove the thyme and serve beef fillet with the broccoli and sprinkled with the lime cooking sauce.

Beef with ginger and courgettes

Servings: 4 I Prep time: 10 minutes I Cook time: 20 minutes
Nutrition facts per serving: calories: 410; carbs: 2 gr; protein: 40 gr; fat: 5 gr.

Ingredients
- ✓ 4 beef fillets (150 gr about for each)
- ✓ 1 lemon
- ✓ 2 courgettes
- ✓ 1/2 shallot
- ✓ 1 tbsp of powdered ginger
- ✓ Olive oil, salt and pepper

Directions
- ➢ First, peel courgettes, then wash and dry it.
- ➢ Cut it little cubes.
- ➢ Peel and wash the shallot too. Dry it and then chop it.
- ➢ Take a non-stick pan and heat the oil.
- ➢ When it is hot, add the courgettes and brown it for 4 minutes, seasoning with salt and italian seasoning.
- ➢ Add water and let cook for other 10 minutes or until water will be absorbed.
- ➢ Let courgettes drain.
- ➢ Wash and dry the fillet and then cut it into small pieces.
- ➢ Wash and dry the lemon, grate the peel, and set it aside and then squeeze the pulp and strain the juice into a bowl.

➤ Put the meat, salt, pepper, olive oil, ginger, and a bit of chopped coriander in the bowl with the lime juice.
➤ Stir gently to mix everything.
➤ Let sauté the beef filet with the sauce for few minutes in a pan.
➤ When it will be done, serve the meat in the centre of the plate.
➤ Add the courgettes cubes and serve.

Cabbage veal

Servings: 4 I Prep time: 5 minutes I Cook time: 40 minutes
Nutrition facts *per serving*: calories: 360; carbs: 5 gr; protein: 35 gr; fat: 4 gr.

Ingredients
✓ 600 gr of lean veal fillet
✓ 400 gr of green cabbage
✓ 1 garlic
✓ 1 bay leaf
✓ 80 ml of beef broth
✓ Olive oil, salt and pepper

Directions
➤ Start with the veal meat. Remove the excess fat then wash and dry it.
➤ Place the rack on a sheet of aluminium foil, brush the veal fillet with a little olive oil and then close the aluminium foil.
➤ Place the veal on a baking sheet.
➤ Bake in the oven at 180ºc for 20 minutes about.
➤ Meanwhile, prepare the cabbage.
➤ Peel, wash and then finely chop the garlic.
➤ Wash the cabbage, dry it, and then cut it into thin slices.
➤ In a pan, put a drizzle of oil to heat. When the oil is hot, sauté chopped garlic for a couple of minutes, stirring constantly to keep it from burning.
➤ Now add the cabbage, season with salt and pepper and mix.
➤ After a couple of minutes, add the broth.
➤ Cook for 30 minutes, adding water if necessary, and stirring occasionally.
➤ As soon as the veal is cooked, remove it from the oven, let the meat rest for 5 minutes and then slice it.
➤ Put the cabbage on the bottom of the serving dish, then over beef slices and sprinkle everything with the cooking juices of the cabbage.

Courgette broth veal

Servings: 4 I Prep time: 15 minutes I Cook time: 15 minutes
Nutrition facts *per serving*: calories: 350; carbs: 4 gr; protein: 23 gr; fat: 11 gr.

Ingredients
✓ 2 slices of lean veal of 120 gr for each
✓ 1 courgette
✓ 300 ml of vegetable stock
✓ 4 tbsp of almond flour
✓ 1 onion
✓ Olive oil, salt and pepper

Directions
➤ First, peel the onion and then chop it.
➤ Peel the courgettes, wash it, and then cut it into slices.
➤ Wash and dry the veal slices and then season with salt and pepper.
➤ Put the almond flour on a plate and then flour the slices and set aside.
➤ Heat a tbsp of oil in a pan and brown the onion for a couple of minutes.
➤ Now add the courgettes and sauté them for a couple of minutes.
➤ Season with salt and pepper, remove the courgettes and put the meat.
➤ Brown the veal meat for 4 minutes per side and then put the courgettes back.
➤ Add the broth and continue cooking for another 4 minutes.
➤ Put the slices and courgettes on serving plates, sprinkle with the cooking juices and serve.

Mozzarella and tomatoes beef

Servings: 4 I Prep time: 10 minutes I Cook time: 20 minutes
Nutrition facts *per serving*: calories: 345; carbs: 3.4 gr protein: 34 gr fat: 2 gr.

Ingredients
✓ 4 slices of lean beef (100 gr for each)
✓ 8 cherry tomatoes
✓ 2 mozzarellas
✓ 1 tsp of dried oregano
✓ Olive oil, salt and pepper to taste

Directions
➤ Start with the beef slices.
➤ Wash them quickly under running water, dry with towel paper and set them aside.
➤ Take a baking dish and lightly brush it with a bit of olive oil.
➤ Now flour the slices of meat and then place them in the pan.

- Wash and dry cherry tomatoes and then cut them into slices.
- Cut the mozzarella into slices too.
- In a bowl, mix together 2 tablespoons of olive oil, salt, pepper and oregano.
- Spread the tomato slices on each slice of meat.
- Sprinkle a little salt and pepper on the tomatoes and then cover with the mozzarella slices.
- Put all ingredients into a baking pan.
- Preheat the oven to 190°c and, once temperature is reached, let cook pizza beef for 15/18 minutes.
- Check the cooking and if they still don't seem cooked, continue for another 2 minutes.
- Serve your mozzarella and tomatoes beef still hot.

Mushrooms and pine nuts beef

Servings: 4 I Prep time: 10 minutes I Cook time: 20 minutes
Nutrition facts per serving: calories: 370; carbs: 1 gr; protein: 39 gr; fat: 8 gr.

Ingredients
- 4 beef fillets of 150 gr for each
- 300 gr of champignon mushrooms
- 4 tbsp of toasted and chopped pine nuts
- ½ shallot
- Olive oil, salt and pepper to taste

Directions
- Start by cleaning the champignon mushrooms.
- Remove any earthy part, wash them well under running water, dry them and then cut them into thin slices.
- Clean the beef filet.
- Remove the excess fat and then wash it under running water and dry it with a paper towel.
- Peel and wash the shallot, then chop it.
- Heat the oil in a pan. As soon as it is hot enough, fry the shallot.
- As soon as the garlic has taken on a golden colour, put the beef in the pan.
- Cook the fillet for 3 minutes on both sides, making sure to seal the meat well.
- Season with salt and pepper.
- After the cook time, put the fillet to rest so that it remains warm anyway.
- In the same pan where you browned the fillets, now cook the mushrooms.
- Cook them for 5 minutes, stirring occasionally, then add the salt and pepper and cook for another 10 minutes.
- Meanwhile, finely chop the toasted pine nuts.
- When the mushrooms are ready, take 4 serving dishes, place one fillet per plate, surround with

the mushrooms and sprinkle them with the mushroom sauce.
- Finish garnishing with the chopped pine nuts and serve.

Mushroom spicy sauce veal

Servings: 4 I Prep time: 10 minutes I Cook time: 20 minutes
Nutrition facts per serving: calories: 380; carbs: 4 gr; protein: 36 gr; fat: 7 gr.

Ingredients
- 600 gr of veal fillet
- 400 gr of mushrooms
- 100 ml of cooking cream
- 1 garlic clove
- 1 tsp mix of onion powder
- Olive oil, salt and pepper

Directions
- First, peel and wash the garlic.
- Remove any earthy part of the mushrooms, wash them under running water, dry them and then cut them into slices.
- Clean the veal fillet. Remove excess fat and then cut into two slices. Wash it and dry with a paper towel.
- Heat the olive oil in a pan. As soon as it is hot, brown the garlic and then remove it.
- Place the beef slices and brown them on both sides until they are well cooked. Season with salt and pepper and mix of spices.
- Remove the beef and keep it warm.
- Now add the mushrooms to the pan where you cooked the beef before. Brown them for 10 minutes and then add the cooking cream and onion powder.
- Stir to mix well,
- Let the sauce reduce and then season with salt and pepper. Add the veal fillet, let it flavour and then turn off the heat.
- Serve the fillet sprinkled with the mushroom sauce.

Olives roasted beef

Servings: 4 I Prep time: 10 minutes I Cook time: 50 minutes
Nutrition facts per serving: calories: 420; carbs: 6.7 gr; protein: 36 gr; fat: 11 gr.

Ingredients
- 600 gr of beef fillet

- ✓ 2 tbsp of green olives
- ✓ 4 dried cherry tomatoes
- ✓ 1 shallot
- ✓ 1 glass of apple cider vinegar
- ✓ Olive oil, salt and pepper

Directions
- ➢ First, peel and wash shallot and then chop it.
- ➢ Dab the dried tomatoes with a paper towel and then chop them.
- ➢ Remove the stone from the olives and then chop them.
- ➢ Put the tomatoes, shallot, and olives in a bowl. Add salt and pepper and mix everything well.
- ➢ Wash and dry the beef meat, remove the excess fat, and then brush it with olive oil.
- ➢ Massage the entire surface of the meat with the chopped tomatoes and olives.
- ➢ Heat two tablespoons of olive oil in a saucepan and brown the meat for two minutes on each side.
- ➢ Add the vinegar, reduce the heat to a minimum and cover the pot with a lid.
- ➢ Continue cooking for another 45 minutes, adding a little water during cooking if necessary.
- ➢ Meanwhile, wash and dry some parsley leaves and then chop them.
- ➢ Once cooked, turn off and let the meat rest for a couple of minutes.
- ➢ Put the roast on a cutting board and cut it into slices.
- ➢ Put the beef roast on serving plates. Sprinkle with the cooking sauce and serve the beef.

Shallots and basil baked beef

Servings: 4 I Prep time: 15 minutes I Cook time: 40 minutes
Nutrition facts per serving: calories: 420; carbs: 5.8 gr; protein: 38 gr; fat: 7 gr.

Ingredients
- ✓ 600 gr of lean beef fillet
- ✓ 4 shallots
- ✓ 10 chopped basil leaves
- ✓ 2 sprigs of rosemary
- ✓ Olive oil, salt and pepper to taste

Directions
- ➢ First, peel and wash the shallots and leave them whole.
- ➢ Bring a pot of water and salt to a boil. When it starts to boil, blanch the shallots for 3 minutes.
- ➢ Once cooked, drain, and set aside.
- ➢ Wash and dry the beef fillet.

- ➢ Heat two tablespoons of olive oil in a pan and, when hot, brown the fillet, two minutes per side.
- ➢ Brush a baking pan with olive oil. Put the fillet with all the cooking juices inside and then add the shallots.
- ➢ Season with oil, salt, and pepper.
- ➢ Wash and dry rosemary sprig and then put them in the baking pan.
- ➢ Wash and chop basil leaves too, then add to the beef.
- ➢ Place the baking pan in the oven and bake at 170°c for 35 minutes.
- ➢ After cooking, remove the baking pan from the oven and place the roast on a cutting board.
- ➢ Cut the roast into slices and place them on serving plates.
- ➢ Add the shallots, sprinkle with parsley and cooking juices and serve.

Spicy beef with fennels

Servings: 4 I Prep time: 10 minutes I Cook time: 20 minutes
Nutrition facts per serving: calories: 355; carbs: 1 gr protein: 38 gr; fat: 4 gr.

Ingredients
- ✓ 600 gr of beef fillet
- ✓ 1 tsp of smoked paprika
- ✓ 1 pinch of chilli powder
- ✓ 2 large fennels
- ✓ 1 tbsp of fennel seeds
- ✓ Olive oil, salt and pepper

Directions
- ➢ Start with the fennels.
- ➢ Remove the inner part, separate the various leaves, wash them under running water, dry them and then cut the fennel into slices.
- ➢ Also wash some pieces of fennel and set them aside.
- ➢ Take a pan and heat half a tablespoon of oil.
- ➢ Let the oil heat up and then put the fennel slices for about ten minutes to sauté, adding salt and a drop of water.
- ➢ Now switch to the beef fillet.
- ➢ Wash it under running water and let it dy.
- ➢ Now take a pan and put 2 sheets of parchment paper inside the pan.
- ➢ Grease the parchment paper with a little oil, add the beef, salt it, sprinkle it with chilli powder and paprika.
- ➢ Then sprinkle beef with a bit of lemon juice and a drizzle of olive oil and the fennel pieces that you had set aside.

➢ Put the beef in a preheated oven at 190° c for about 15 minutes.
➢ As soon as they are ready, remove the beef fillet from the parchment paper, remove the fennel pieces too and place beef in a serving dish surrounded by previously cooked fennel.
➢ Sprinkle with fennel seeds and serve your beef dish still hot.

Vinegar and mustard veal fillet

Servings: 4 I Prep time: 3 hours marinated I Cook time: 20 minutes
Nutrition facts per serving: calories: 370; carbs: 4 gr; protein: 36 gr; fat: 2 gr.

Ingredients
✓ 600 gr of lean veal fillet
✓ 100 ml of apple cider vinegar
✓ 60 ml of mustard
✓ 1 tbsp of nutmeg
✓ Olive oil
✓ Salt and pepper to taste

Directions
➢ Start the recipe by quickly washing veal fillet and let it dry.
➢ Meanwhile, mix the olive oil, vinegar, a pinch of nutmeg and mustard.
➢ Mix them well together to obtain a marinade.
➢ Clean and wash the veal fillet.
➢ Put the cleaned veal fillet directly into the marinade.
➢ Cover it with cling film and leave it to marinate in the fridge for at least 3 hours.
➢ Remove it from the fridge and wait for the meat to reach room temperature.
➢ Preheat the oven at 200°c.
➢ Once temperature is reached, place the marinated veal in a baking pan.
➢ Put the baking pan in the preheated oven and let cook for 20 minutes about.
➢ As soon as cooked, slice veal fillet.
➢ Season the meat with salt and pepper and serve.

Pork recipes

***

Blue cheese sauce pork loin

Servings: 4 I Prep time: 10 minutes I Cook time: 60 minutes

Nutrition facts per serving: calories: 410; carbs: 2 gr; protein: 31 gr; fat: 14 gr.

Ingredients
✓ 600 gr of whole pork tenderloin
✓ 1 sprig of rosemary
✓ 1 glass of cooking cream
✓ 100 gr of blue cheese
✓ Olive oil, salt and pepper to taste

Directions
➢ First, wash and dry the pork fillet and then sprinkle the entire surface of the meat with salt and pepper.
➢ Cut the fillet into 8 slices of the same size.
➢ Wash the sprig of rosemary and divide it into four parts.
➢ Put the rosemary between the meat.
➢ Brush the surface of the meat with olive oil and then put it in a baking pan brushed with olive oil.
➢ Cook the fillets at 190°c for 20 minutes, then turn the fillets and continue cooking for another 35 minutes.
➢ Once cooked, remove the baking pan from the oven and let the meat rest for 10 minutes.
➢ Then move on to prepare the blue cheese sauce.
➢ Cut the gorgonzola into cubes and put it in a saucepan with the cooking cream.
➢ Put the saucepan on the stove and cook until the blue cheese has completely melted, and the sauce has taken on a thick and homogeneous consistency.
➢ At this point, put the meat on a cutting board, and cut the pork loin into slices.
➢ Put the meat on serving plates, sprinkle them with the blue cheese sauce and serve.

Broccoli and cheddar pork roll

Servings: 4 I Prep time: 40 minutes I Cook time: 60 minutes
Nutrition facts per serving: calories: 390; carbs: 5.8 gr; protein: 30 gr; fat: 11 gr.

Ingredients
✓ 600 gr of pork loin
✓ 350 gr of broccoli flowers
✓ 100 gr of cubed cheddar
✓ 20 ml of olive oil
✓ Salt and pepper to taste.

Directions
➢ First, wash the broccoli flowers under running water and then dry them.
➢ Then put them in a pot with water and salt and cook for 20 minutes.

➤ While broccoli florets are cooking, take the pork loin, remove the bones and fat, and then cut it horizontally in half.
➤ Beat it with a meat mallet to soften and thin it, then sprinkle it on both sides with salt and pepper.
➤ When the broccoli is cooked, drain it, let it cool and then cut it into small pieces.
➤ Take a sheet of cling film and place pork loin on top.
➤ Place the broccoli first and then the cubed cheddar inside the pork.
➤ Roll up everything, using the plastic wrap and let it rest in the fridge for 30 minutes.
➤ Meanwhile, preheat the oven to 180° c.
➤ Brush a pan with olive oil and lie inside the roll.
➤ Cook for 30 minutes, adding a little water if necessary.
➤ Remove from the oven, let it rest for 5 minutes and then cut the pork roll into slices and serve.

Citrus fruit and rosemary pork loin

Servings: 4 I Prep time: 20 minutes I Cook time: 55 minutes
Nutrition facts per serving: calories: 390; carbs: 6 gr; protein: 30 gr; fat: 5 gr.

Ingredients
✓ 600 gr of pork tenderloin
✓ 2 oranges
✓ 1 lemon
✓ 1 sprig of rosemary
✓ Olive oil, salt and pepper to taste

Directions
➤ Start the preparation by washing and drying the pork tenderloin. Remove excess fat from the meat.
➤ Wash oranges and lemon and then grate the peel and cut the pulp into cubes.
➤ Wash and dry, rosemary sprig.
➤ Brush a baking pan with olive oil and then put the meat inside.
➤ Put the lemon and orange pulp inside.
➤ Add rosemary too.
➤ Season with oil, salt and pepper, sprinkle with the grated citrus peel and place in the oven.
➤ Bake at 170°c for 50 minutes, then remove the baking pan and let it rest for 5 minutes.
➤ Mash the lemon and orange pulp and then cut the meat into slices.
➤ Put the meat on serving plates, sprinkle with the cooking juices and serve.

Courgettes and tomatoes pork loin

Servings: 4 I Prep time: 10+60 minutes of marinating I Cook time: 20 minutes
Nutrition facts per serving: calories: 240; carbs: 4.8 gr; protein: 25 gr; fat: 9 gr.

Ingredients:
✓ 400 gr of pork loin
✓ 2 courgettes
✓ 4 cherry tomatoes
✓ The juice of half a lemon
✓ Olive oil, salt and pepper

Directions
➤ Wash and dry the pork loin and remove excess fat.
➤ Put the pork in a baking dish.
➤ Season it with lemon juice, salt, pepper, thyme, and a tablespoon of olive oil.
➤ Cover the baking dish with cling film and marinate for 1 hour at room temperature.
➤ Meanwhile, wash the courgettes and cut them into thin slices.
➤ Wash and dry the cherry tomatoes and then cut them into 4 parts.
➤ Heat a grill and when it is hot, put the courgettes to grill.
➤ Grill them for 4 minutes on each side and then set them aside on a plate.
➤ Now go on to cook the pork loin. Put it on the grill and cook for 10 minutes per side.
➤ Once cooked, remove the pork from the grill and place it on a cutting board.
➤ Cut it into thin strips and then put it in a bowl.
➤ Also cut the courgettes into small pieces and place them in the bowl with the pork loin.
➤ Finally add the cherry tomatoes and season with oil, salt, and pepper.
➤ Combine well all ingredients and serve.

Ginger pork loin

Servings: 4 I Prep time: 10 minutes + 2hours marinating I Cook time: 20 minutes
Nutrition facts per serving: calories: 320; carbs: 2 gr; protein: 30 gr; fat: 4 gr.

Ingredients
✓ 1 pork fillet of 600 gr
✓ 2 tablespoons of low-carb soy sauce
✓ 2 tablespoons of olive oil
✓ 1 tablespoon of grated ginger
✓ Salt and pepper to taste

Directions

➢ Start by eliminating the excess fat from the fillet and cut into pieces about 2 cm thick by cutting them lengthwise.
➢ Wash and dry the fillets.
➢ In a bowl put the soy sauce, and ginger. Stir until the sauce has melted slightly.
➢ Now add the olive oil, salt, pepper, and mix.
➢ Now put the pork fillets inside the bowl and leave to marinate for 2 hours.
➢ When 2 hours has passed, preheat your over to 210° c.
➢ Put the fillets in the oven and cook them for 15/20 minutes.
➢ Turn them every 5 minutes and brush them with the marinating liquid.
➢ As soon as they are cooked, remove them from the oven and let them rest for 5 minutes.
➢ Put the marinade in a saucepan and let it reduce by half.
➢ Put the fillets on plates, sprinkle them with the marinating liquid and serve.

Grilled pork chop

Servings: 4 I Prep time: 10 minutes + 30 minutes of marinating I Cook time: 20 minutes
Nutrition facts per serving: calories: 390; carbs: 1 gr; protein: 24 gr; fat: 16 gr.

Ingredients for 4servings
✓ 4 pork chops of 100 gr each
✓ 1 clove of garlic
✓ 2 sprigs of thyme
✓ Olive oil, salt and pepper to taste

Directions
➢ Wash and dry the thyme sprigs, remove the needles, and then chop them.
➢ Peel and wash the garlic and then chop it.
➢ Wash and dry the chops and remove all excess fat.
➢ Put the chops in a baking dish and season with oil, salt, pepper, rosemary, and garlic.
➢ Cover the bowl with cling film and marinate for 30 minutes.
➢ After 30 minutes, heat a grill and, when it is hot, put the chops to grill.
➢ Cook for 10 minutes on each side and then remove them from the grill.
➢ Put the chops on serving plates, brush them with a little marinade and serve.

Hazelnut sauce pork fillet

Servings: 4 I Prep time: 10 minutes I Cook time: 55 minutes
Nutrition facts per serving: calories: 340; carbs: 6.8 gr; protein: 30 gr; fat:10 gr.

Ingredients
✓ 1 whole pork fillet of 600 gr
✓ 4 tbsp of chopped hazelnuts
✓ 1 glass of cooking cream
✓ 1 glass of apple cider vinegar
✓ 1 shallot
✓ Olive oil, salt and pepper to taste

Directions
➢ First, peel and wash the shallot.
➢ Remove the excess fat from the pork tenderloin and then wash it and pat it dry with a paper towel.
➢ Rub the entire surface of the meat with shallot, then brush it with oil, and season with salt and pepper.
➢ Put the fillet in a baking pan brushed with olive oil and cook at 170°c for 55 minutes.
➢ Turn and brush the meat with oil every 10 minutes.
➢ As soon as it is cooked, remove it from the oven and let it rest for 10 minutes.
➢ Meanwhile, make the hazelnut sauce.
➢ Put a tablespoon of olive oil in a pan and as soon as it is hot enough add the chopped hazelnuts.
➢ Sauté 2 minutes, and then add the vinegar.
➢ Mix, let the wine evaporate and then add the cooking cream.
➢ Let the sauce thicken, season with salt and pepper and turn off.
➢ Now cut the fillet into slices.
➢ Put the slices of fillet on plates, sprinkle the whole surface of the meat with the hazelnut sauce and serve.

Lime and garlic pork ribs

Servings: 4 I Prep time: 10 minutes + 2 hours of marinating I Cook time: 2 hours
Nutrition facts per serving: calories: 380; carbs: 1 gr; protein: 24 gr; fat:14 gr.

Ingredients
✓ 500 gr of pork ribs
✓ 4 cloves of garlic
✓ 4 limes
✓ 500 ml of meat broth
✓ Olive oil, salt and pepper to taste

Directions

➤ First peel and wash the garlic cloves and then chop them.
➤ Wash and dry the limes. Grate the zest and strain the juice into a bowl.
➤ Wash and dry the pork tips and then put them in a bowl.
➤ Season with lime zest and juice, minced garlic, 4 tablespoons of olive oil, salt, and pepper.
➤ Stir to flavour the meat well.
➤ Cover the bowl with cling film and leave to marinate for 2 hours.
➤ After 2 hours, pour 3 tablespoons of oil into a pan.
➤ When it is hot enough, put the tacks to brown.
➤ Now add the meat broth and the marinating liquid.
➤ Cover the pan with the lid and cook for 2 hours, stirring often.
➤ After cooking, turn off and put the pins in the serving dishes.
➤ Sprinkle with the cooking juices and serve.

Mustard seeds pork loin

Servings: 4 I Prep time: 10 minutes I Cook time: 20 minutes
Nutrition facts per serving: calories: 225; carbs: 1 gr; protein: 31 gr; fat: 9 gr.

Ingredients
✓ 4 slices of pork tenderloin (100 gr for each)
✓ 2 tbsp of mustard seeds
✓ Olive oil to taste
✓ Salt and pepper to taste

Directions
➤ First, wash and dry the pork tenderloin.
➤ Heat a tablespoon of olive oil in a pan.
➤ When the oil is hot, add the mustard seeds and sauté them for a couple of minutes.
➤ Now add the pork fillet and brown it for a couple of minutes on each side.
➤ Season with salt and pepper and turn off.
➤ Brush a baking dish with olive oil and put the pork fillet inside.
➤ Sprinkle with the cooking juices left in the pan and place the baking dish in the oven.
➤ Cook at 190° c for 10 minutes.
➤ Once cooked, remove the baking dish from the oven and let it rest for a couple of minutes.
➤ Put the pork loin on the plate, sprinkle with the cooking juices and serve.

Orange pork skewers

Servings: 4 I Prep time: 10 minutes + 6 hours of marinating I Cook time: 10 minutes
Nutrition facts per serving: calories: 300; carbs: 2 gr; protein: 24 gr; fat: 10 gr.

Ingredients
✓ 400 gr of pork tenderloin
✓ 2 oranges
✓ 3 tablespoons of apple cider vinegar
✓ 2 cloves of garlic
✓ Olive oil, salt and pepper to taste

Directions
➤ Wash and dry the pork tenderloin. Remove all excess fat, cut it into cubes and put it in a bowl.
➤ Peel and wash the garlic cloves and then chop them.
➤ Put the garlic, filtered orange juice, apple cider vinegar, salt, pepper, and olive oil in the bowl with the meat.
➤ Mix well and then cover the bowl with cling film.
➤ Put the bowl in the fridge and marinate for 6 hours.
➤ After marinating, remove the bowl from the fridge and start skewered the meat.
➤ When all the skewers are ready, reheat a grill and, when it is hot, put the skewers to grill.
➤ Cook for 3 minutes on each side, then remove them from the grill and place them on serving plates.
➤ Sprinkle with the filtered marinating liquid and serve.

Paprika flavoured pork loin

Servings: 4 I Prep time: 10 minutes I Cook time: 15 minutes
Nutrition facts per serving: calories: 310; carbs: 2 gr; protein: 32 gr; fat: 6 gr.

Ingredients
✓ 4 slices of pork loin (150 gr for each)
✓ 1 tsp of paprika
✓ 1 garlic clove
✓ Almond flour, just enough
✓ 2 glasses of vegetable broth
✓ Olive, salt and pepper

Directions
➤ First, peel and wash the garlic and then chop it.
➤ Put a bit of almond flour on a plate and add salt and pepper.
➤ Mix well and then pass the pork slices on the flour.
➤ Heat a tablespoon of olive oil in a pan.
➤ When the oil is hot, add the garlic and brown it.

- ➤ Add the pork slices and cook 1 minute per side.
- ➤ Now add the broth and paprika.
- ➤ Cook for another 5 minutes, then season with salt and pepper and turn off.
- ➤ Put the meat on the plate. Sprinkle it with the cooking sauce and serve.

Pecans and cheddar crusted pork loin

Servings: 4 I Prep time: 10 minutes I Cook time: 20 minutes
Nutrition facts per serving: calories: 360; carbs: 2 gr; protein: 32 gr; fat: 7 gr.

Ingredients
- ✓ 4 slices of pork loin (100 gr for each)
- ✓ 2 sage leaves
- ✓ 40 gr of chopped pecans
- ✓ 40 gr of grated cheddar
- ✓ Olive oil, salt and pepper to taste

Directions
- ➤ First, start with the pork loin.
- ➤ Remove the excess fat and then if the slices are not thin enough, thin them with a meat mallet.
- ➤ Wash and dry the pork slices with a paper towel and then sprinkle them on both sides with salt and pepper.
- ➤ Wash and dry the sage.
- ➤ Place the 4 pork slices on a cutting board, place 2 sage leaves inside.
- ➤ Close the slices with the remaining slices, sealing them with toothpicks.
- ➤ Mix together the chopped pecans with the grated cheddar cheese.
- ➤ Pass the slices over the pecans and cheddar flour, pressing them to make the breading adhere well.
- ➤ Heat the olive oil in a pan and as soon as it is hot, put the pork loin to brown.
- ➤ Turn them over and cook until the meat is well cooked and golden on the outside.
- ➤ Serve the crusted pork loin immediately and hot, sprinkled with the cooking juices.

Parmesan and almond pork loin

Servings: 4 I Prep time: 10 minutes I Cook time: 15 minutes
Nutrition facts per serving: calories: 390; carbs: 2 gr; protein: 34 gr; fat: 14 gr.

Ingredients
- ✓ 4 slices of pork loin of 100 gr each

- ✓ 2 eggs
- ✓ 60 gr of almond flour
- ✓ 50 gr of grated parmesan cheese
- ✓ 1 tsp of fresh parsley
- ✓ Olive oil, salt and pepper

Directions
- ➤ First, rinse the pork loin under running water and pat it dry with absorbent paper. Remove all excess fat.
- ➤ Wash and finely chop parsley.
- ➤ Shell the eggs in a bowl. Add salt and pepper and beat them with a fork.
- ➤ Dip the loin slices in the eggs.
- ➤ Put the almond flour, parmesan, and a bit of parsley on a plate.
- ➤ Mix well and then pass the slices of loin in the breading.
- ➤ Press the meat firmly onto the breading to ensure that it covers the entire surface of the meat.
- ➤ Pour three tablespoons of oil into a pan.
- ➤ When the oil is hot, put the cutlets to cook. Cook for 7-8 minutes per side, until, in practice, the outer surface of the meat is golden brown.
- ➤ After cooking, dab the meat with absorbent paper to remove all excess oil.
- ➤ Now put the pork loin on the serving plates and serve.

Walnuts pork loin

Servings: 4 I Prep time: 10 minutes I Cook time: 20 minutes
Nutrition facts per serving: calories: 395; carbs: 2 gr; protein: 34 gr; fat: 15 gr.

Ingredients
- ✓ 4 slices of pork loin of 100 gr each
- ✓ 2 eggs
- ✓ Almond flour, just enough
- ✓ 2 tbsp of chopped walnuts
- ✓ Olive oil, salt and pepper

Directions
- ➤ Start by rinsing the pork loin under running water and pat it dry with a paper towel. Remove all excess fat.
- ➤ Shell the eggs in a bowl. Add salt and pepper and beat them with a fork.
- ➤ Dip the loin slices in the eggs.
- ➤ Put the almond flour and walnuts on a plate.
- ➤ Mix well and then pass the slices of loin in the breading.
- ➤ Press the meat firmly onto the breading to ensure that it covers the entire surface of the meat.
- ➤ Pour three tablespoons of oil into a pan.

- ➢ When the oil is hot, put the cutlets to cook. Cook for 7-8 minutes per side, until, in practice, the outer surface of the meat is golden brown.
- ➢ After cooking, dab the meat with a paper towel to remove all excess oil.
- ➢ Now put the cutlets on the serving plates and serve.

Yellow pepper and sage pork fillets

Servings: 4 I Prep time: 15 minutes I Cook time: 50 minutes
Nutrition facts per serving: calories: 390; carbs: 5 gr; protein: 30 gr; fat: 7 gr.

Ingredients
- ✓ 4 pork fillets of 120 gr for each
- ✓ 1 glass of apple cider vinegar
- ✓ 2 sage leaves
- ✓ 2 yellow peppers
- ✓ Olive oil, salt and pepper

Directions
- ➢ First wash and dry the pork fillets and then remove, if there is, any excess fat.
- ➢ Remove the stalk from the yellow peppers. Clean them and remove all internal seeds and filaments.
- ➢ Cut yellow peppers into little strips.
- ➢ In a bowl, mix together the apple cider vinegar and 4 tablespoons of olive oil.
- ➢ Brush the entire surface of the meat with the emulsion and then sprinkle it with salt and pepper.
- ➢ Brush a baking pan with olive oil and put the meat inside.
- ➢ Wash and dry sage.
- ➢ Put sage, in the pan with the pork fillet.
- ➢ Sprinkle with yellow pepper strips and put the baking pan in the oven.
- ➢ Cook at 170° c for 50 minutes.
- ➢ Once cooked, remove the pan from the oven and let the meat rest for 5 minutes.
- ➢ Cut the pork fillet into slices and place it on serving plates.
- ➢ Sprinkle with the cooking juices and serve.

Lamb recipes

***

Artichokes and rosemary leg of lamb

Servings: 4 I Prep time: 20 minutes I Cook time: 30 minutes
Nutrition facts per serving: calories: 350, carbs: 6 gr; protein: 27 gr; fat: 12 gr.

Ingredients
- ✓ A leg of boneless and fatless lamb of 800 gr
- ✓ 4 artichokes
- ✓ 2 tbsp of wine
- ✓ 4 rosemary sprigs
- ✓ Olive oil, salt and pepper to taste

Directions
- ➢ First remove the stem, the harder outer leaves, then cut them into 4 parts and remove the inner beard.
- ➢ Wash and dry some rosemary leaves and chop them.
- ➢ Put a tablespoon of olive oil in a pan and as soon as it is hot, add the artichokes and half a glass of water.
- ➢ Stir, season with salt and pepper and cook for 15 minutes.
- ➢ Wash and dry the thyme.
- ➢ Wash and dry the leg of lamb and then cut it in half.
- ➢ Sprinkle the inside of the meat with salt and pepper rosemary and wine and then add the filling.
- ➢ Roll it up and secure it with kitchen twine.
- ➢ Brush the surface of the meat with olive oil and place it in a baking pan brushed with olive oil
- ➢ Cook at 160°c for 15 minutes and then turn the meat.
- ➢ Raise the temperature to 190° v and continue cooking for another 10 minutes.
- ➢ After Cook time, remove the lamb from the oven and let it rest for 5 minutes.
- ➢ Now cut the lamb into slices, put them on serving plates with artichokes and serve.

Basil sauce lamb chops

Servings: 4 I Prep time: 15 minutes I Cook time: 15 minutes
Nutrition facts per serving: calories: 360; carbs: 1 gr; protein: 32 gr; fat: 16 gr.

Ingredients
- ✓ 4 lamb chops (150 gr for each)
- ✓ 10 basil leaves
- ✓ 1 clove of garlic
- ✓ Olive oil, salt and pepper

Directions

➢ First, peel and wash the garlic clove and then chop it.
➢ Wash and dry the basil leaves.
➢ Wash and dry the lamb chops and remove excess fat.
➢ Heat a tablespoon of olive oil in a pan.
➢ When it is hot, add the garlic and basil and cook for a couple of minutes.
➢ Now add the lamb chops and brown them for 3 minutes per side.
➢ Season with salt and pepper and turn off.
➢ Brush a baking pan with olive oil and put the chops inside.
➢ Place the baking pan in the oven and bake at 200° c for 10 minutes.
➢ In the meantime, put the cooking juices in the glass of the blender, add a little olive oil and blend until you get a thick and homogeneous sauce.
➢ After cooking, remove the lamb from the oven and let it rest for a couple of minutes.
➢ Put the lamb on the plate, sprinkle with the basil sauce and serve.

Bell peppers and paprika lamb

Servings: 4 I Prep time: 15 minutes I Cook time: 20 minutes
Nutrition facts per serving: calories: 400; carbs: 6 gr; protein: 28 gr; fat: 12 gr.

Ingredients
✓ 1 rack of lamb of 800 gr
✓ 2 red bell peppers
✓ 1 glass of red wine
✓ 1 tsp of smoked paprika
✓ 60 gr of almond flour
✓ 1 garlic glove
✓ Olive oil, salt and pepper

Directions
➢ First, wash and dry the rack and then cut it into small pieces.
➢ Remove the caps from the peppers, remove the seeds and white filaments and then wash them. Cut them into strips.
➢ Peel and wash a garlic clove and then chop it.
➢ Put the almond flour on a plate with a little salt and pepper, paprika and mix it.
➢ Dip the lamb pieces in paprika almond flour.
➢ Brush a baking pan with a little oil and place the pieces of loin inside.
➢ Add the red bell peppers, chopped garlic, and then season everything with oil, salt and pepper.

➢ Sprinkle with the wine and then put the baking pan in the oven.
➢ Cook at 180°c for 10 minutes. Then turn the lamb.
➢ Bake for another 10 minutes and then remove the baking pan from the oven.
➢ Put the pieces of lamb on the plates, garnish with the peppers and serve.

Onion and parsley leg of lamb

Servings: 4 I Prep time: 20 minutes I Cook time: 20 minutes
Nutrition facts per serving: calories: 340; carbs: 2.2 gr; protein: 24 gr; fat: 9 gr.

Ingredients
✓ A leg of boneless lamb, 600 gr
✓ 2 onions, chopped
✓ 1 bunch of fresh chopped parsley
✓ ½ glass of red wine
✓ Olive oil, salt and pepper

Directions
➢ Wash,dry and chop the parsley.
➢ Put a tablespoon of olive oil in a pan and as soon as it is hot, add the onions and parsley, and half a glass of water.
➢ Stir, season with salt and pepper and cook for 15 minutes.
➢ Meanwhile, wash and dry the leg of lamb and then cut it in half.
➢ Sprinkle the inside of the meat with salt and pepper and the red wine and then add the filling.
➢ Roll it up and secure it with kitchen twine.
➢ Brush the surface of the meat with olive oil and place it in a baking pan brushed with olive oil.
➢ Cook at 190° for 15/20 minutes and then turn the meat.
➢ After cook time, remove the lamb from the oven and let it rest for 5 minutes.
➢ Now cut the lamb into slices, put them on serving plates with parsley and serve.

Orange and herbs lamb

Servings: 4 I Prep time: 20 minutes I Cook time: 45 minutes
Nutrition facts per serving: calories: 310; carbs: 3 gr; protein: 25 gr; fat: 8 gr.

Ingredients
✓ 800 gr of rack of lamb
✓ 1 tbsp of mixed chopped aromatics herbs

✓ 1 orange
✓ Olive oil, salt and pepper

Directions

➢ First, remove excess fat from the loin, wash it and then dry it.
➢ Wash and dry the orange and grate the zest.
➢ Peel and wash the garlic cloves and then chop them.
➢ Brush a baking pan with olive oil and then put the rack inside.
➢ Season with oil, salt, pepper. Then add the chopped aromatic herbs, garlic, and orange zest.
➢ Cover the baking pan with cling film and put it to marinate in the fridge for 2 hours.
➢ After the two hours, remove the cling film and put the aluminium foil around the bones.
➢ Place the baking pan in the oven and bake at 180°C for 45 minutes.
➢ Once cooked, remove the baking pan from the oven and let the meat rest for a few minutes.
➢ Cut the lamb into slices, put them on a serving dish and serve.

Duck recipes

***

Green pepper sauce duck

Servings: 4 I Prep time: 12 hours I Cook time: 20 minutes
Nutrition facts per serving: calories: 450; carbs: 3; protein: 34; fat: 32.

Ingredients
✓ 2 duck breasts of 300 g each
✓ 1 tbsp of green peppercorns
✓ ½ glass of apple cider vinegar
✓ 120 gr of butter
✓ Oliver oil, salt and pepper to taste

Directions
➢ First, wash and dry the duck breasts and then cut the skin by making horizontal cuts with a knife.
➢ Brush them with oil and season with salt and pepper.
➢ Put the duck breasts in the fridge and marinate for 12 hours.
➢ After 12 hours, remove the duck from the fridge and let it rest for a few minutes at room temperature.
➢ Grease a pan and place it to heat on.

➢ When it is hot, add the butter and let it melt completely.
➢ At this point, add the duck breasts, starting cooking from the skin side.
➢ Cover the oven and cook for 10 minutes, sprinkling the meat with melted butter from time to time.
➢ After 10 minutes, turn the meat and proceed in the same way.
➢ Check the cooking with a cooking thermometer and if the temperature of the meat is 65°c remove it from the oven and place it on a cutting board.
➢ In the meantime, that the meat rests, prepare the sauce.
➢ Put the green pepper in the oven and deglaze with the apple cider vinegar.
➢ When the vinegar has evaporated, remove the oven from the heat.
➢ Now cut the duck breasts into slices and place them on serving plates.
➢ Sprinkle with the green pepper sauce and serve.

Lemon and courgette duck breast

Servings: 4 I Prep time: 10 minutes I Cook time: 50 minutes
Nutrition facts per serving: calories: 390; carbs: 6.8 gr; protein: 21 gr; fat: 25 gr.

Ingredients

✓ 1 duck breast (600 gr about)
✓ 1 courgette
✓ The juice of 1 lemon
✓ 2 glasses of vegetable broth
✓ Olive oil, salt and pepper

Directions
➢ First, place the duck breast in a non-stick saucepan with the skin facing the bottom of the saucepan.
➢ Cover and brown for a few minutes, until it has released a little fat.
➢ Then remove the fat, add a drop of broth, salt and pepper, cover and continue cooking over moderate heat for about 40 minutes, or until pricked with a fork, it is tender.
➢ Meanwhile. Peel, wash and cut courgette into julienne strips.
➢ In another saucepan, sauté the courgette over high heat.
➢ After a few minutes, add the duck breast, sprinkle with the lemon, and let it all flavour together.
➢ You can serve your duck dish with courgette strips and cooking juices.

Orange and cinnamon roasted duck

Servings: 4 I Prep time: 10 minutes I Cook time: 15 minutes
Nutrition facts per serving: calories: 510; carbs: 7 gr; protein: 32 gr; fat: 38 gr.

Ingredients
- ✓ 800 gr of duck breast
- ✓ 1 glass of unsweetened orange juice
- ✓ 2 teaspoons of ground cinnamon
- ✓ Olive oil, salt and pepper

Directions
- ➢ Wash and dry the duck breasts and then cut the skin with a knife.
- ➢ Brush the meat with olive oil and then season with salt and pepper.
- ➢ Grease a pan with a bit of olive oil.
- ➢ When it is hot, place the duck skin side up.
- ➢ Cook for 3 minutes and then turn it over.
- ➢ Cook for another 3 minutes and then turn it skin side again.
- ➢ Deglaze with the orange juice and then cook with the lid on for another 5/6 minutes.
- ➢ When cooked, remove the duck from the heat and let it rest for 5 minutes.
- ➢ Take the duck, put it on a cutting board and cut it into slices.
- ➢ Put the slices of meat on a serving dish, sprinkle with the sauce and serve.

Porcini duck

Servings: 4 I Prep time: 10 minutes I Cook time: 60 minutes
Nutrition facts per serving: calories: 410; carbs: 6 gr; protein: 30 gr; fat: 25 gr.

Ingredients
- ✓ 400 gr of duck breast
- ✓ 400 gr porcini mushrooms
- ✓ 150 gr tomato puree
- ✓ 1 celery
- ✓ 60 ml of cooking cream
- ✓ Salt and pepper

Directions
- ➢ First take the cleaned duck breast and cut it into pieces.
- ➢ Place the duck pieces in a pan and then pass them in the oven at 220°c for about 20 minutes.
- ➢ Meanwhile, clean the porcini mushrooms by gently scraping the stems and rubbing the caps with a damp cloth (or fast passing them under cold water if you prefer), then slicing them into thin slices.

- ➢ Peel and finely chop the celery and onion and a clove of garlic together.
- ➢ Put the mince to dry in a very large saucepan, with 5 tablespoons of oil.
- ➢ Add the prepared mushrooms and brown them then add the duck pieces, which must be in one layer only.
- ➢ Sprinkle the meat with a bit of red wine and after it has partially evaporated, add the tomato puree and as much hot broth as it will be enough to cover the duck pieces.
- ➢ Salt, pepper, cover, and simmer over low heat for about an hour and 45 minutes, stirring the pan from time to time, to make sure that the meat does not stick to the bottom.
- ➢ At the end of cooking, the duck will be tender but not undone; then add the cream and a spoonful of chopped parsley.
- ➢ Leave on the heat for a few more minutes, just enough time for the sauce to thicken, then serve.
- ➢ Serve the duck with the porcini cream.

Teriyaki duck

Servings: 4 I Prep time: 30 minutes marinating I Cook time: 15 minutes
Nutrition facts per serving: calories: 450; carbs: 3.8 gr; protein: 27 gr; fat: 30 gr.

Ingredients
- ✓ 4 duck breasts with the fat part (approx. 220 g each)
- ✓ 1 tbsp of liquid stevia
- ✓ 300 ml of low-carb soy sauce
- ✓ Juice of 3 lemons

Directions
- ➢ First mix the stevia and soy sauce.
- ➢ Add the lemon juice too.
- ➢ Cross the layer of fat on the duck breast.
- ➢ Brush the duck breast on both sides with the marinade, cover it and put it in the fridge for about 30 min.
- ➢ Pat the duck breast dry and cook the remaining marinade in a pan until you have a sauce / until it has the consistency of a syrup.
- ➢ Heat the pan and roast the meat for approx. 5 minutes.
- ➢ To make the fat layer crisp, turn the duck breasts and continue cooking for about 2 more minutes.
- ➢ Sprinkle with the rest of the marinade and serve your duck.

Rabbit recipes

***

Courgette and shallot rabbit

Servings: 4 I Prep time: 15 minutes I Cook time: 50 minutes
Nutrition facts per serving: calories: 320; carbs: 6 gr; protein: 35 gr; fat: 3 gr.

Ingredients
- ✓ 800 gr of rabbit already cut into pieces
- ✓ 1 shallot
- ✓ 2 courgettes
- ✓ 1 glass of vegetable broth
- ✓ ½ glass of white wine
- ✓ Olive oil, salt and pepper

Directions
- ➤ First, peel the shallot, wash it and then chop it.
- ➤ Wash the courgettes, then cut into strips, or cubes.
- ➤ Wash and dry the rabbit pieces.
- ➤ Put them in a food bag and add salt, pepper.
- ➤ Beat the bag well to flour the rabbit well.
- ➤ Grease a pan with olive oil and put it to expire with two tablespoons of olive oil.
- ➤ When the oil is hot enough, add the shallot and cook until it is completely golden.
- ➤ Place the rabbit pieces and brown them on all sides for 10 minutes.
- ➤ Deglaze with half a glass of white wine and let it evaporate.
- ➤ Add the courgettes, mix well, season with salt and pepper, sprinkle with the vegetable broth and cook for 40 minutes.
- ➤ After cooking, remove the rabbit from the heat and place the rabbit and courgettes on serving plates.
- ➤ Sprinkle with the cooking juices and serve.

Mushrooms and onion rabbit

Servings: 4 I Prep time: 15 minutes I Cook time: 60 minutes
Nutrition facts per serving: calories: 300; carbs: 2 gr; protein: 28 gr; fat: 3 gr.

Ingredients
- ✓ 1 rabbit in pieces
- ✓ 300 gr of mushrooms
- ✓ 1 clove of garlic
- ✓ ½ onion
- ✓ 3 sage leaves
- ✓ ½ of glass of white wine
- ✓ Olive oil and salt

Directions
- ➤ First, he must remove all the fatty parts from the rabbit and quickly rinse the pieces.
- ➤ Peel wash and finely chop half an onion after washing it and put it in a pan with three tablespoons of oil.
- ➤ As soon as the onion has heated up, without frying, add the rabbit pieces and the sage leaves.
- ➤ Cook without a lid over medium heat until lightly browned.
- ➤ Season with salt. Add the wine and continue cooking over medium heat with a covered pot, leaving a small vent.
- ➤ Cook for about 60 minutes, turning the pieces occasionally and adding a few ladles of water if necessary.
- ➤ Meanwhile, rinse the mushrooms quickly, drain them well and put them in a pan with a clove of garlic.
- ➤ When the rabbit is almost cooked, add the previously cooked mushrooms and cook together for about ten minutes.
- ➤ Cook for about 15 minutes, deglaze with a drop of wine, and let it evaporate and turn off the heat.
- ➤ You can serve your rabbit with mushrooms.

Mustard and onion rabbit

Servings: 4 I Prep time: 15 minutes I Cook time: 20 minutes
Nutrition facts per serving: calories: 420; carbs: 8 gr; protein: 40 gr; fat: 9 gr.

Ingredients
- ✓ 800 gr of rabbit cut into pieces
- ✓ 1 onion
- ✓ 100 ml of fresh cream
- ✓ 4 tbsp of mustard
- ✓ 600 ml of vegetable broth
- ✓ Olive oil, salt and pepper

Directions
- ➤ Wash the rabbit thoroughly under running water and then pat it dry with a paper towel.
- ➤ Peel and wash the onion and then chop it.
- ➤ Heat a pan with olive oil
- ➤ As soon as the oil starts to sizzle, add the rabbit, and brown it on all sides for 10 minutes.
- ➤ Add a little white wine and let it evaporate.
- ➤ Now add the mustard and the vegetable broth, and season with salt and pepper.
- ➤ Cover with the lid and cook for an hour.

> Once cooked, remove the rabbit, and place it on serving plates.
> Put the cream in the same pot and cook until the sauce has thickened.
> Now sprinkle the rabbit with the sauce and serve.

Rabbit with bell peppers

Servings: 4 I Prep time: 15 minutes I Cook time: 50 minutes
Nutrition facts per serving: calories: 370; carbs: 9 gr; protein: 34 gr; fat: 3 gr.

Ingredients
✓ 800 gr of rabbit already cut into pieces
✓ 1 clove of garlic
✓ 2 red peppers
✓ 1 glass of vegetable broth
✓ 1 glass of white wine
✓ Olive oil, salt and pepper

Directions
> Peel the garlic, wash it, and then chop it.
> Remove the cap, seeds, and white filaments from the peppers. Wash them, dry them, and cut them into strips.
> Wash and dry the rabbit pieces.
> Put them in a food bag and add salt and pepper.
> Grease a pan with olive oil and put it to expire with two tablespoons of olive oil.
> When the oil is hot enough, add the garlic and cook until it is completely golden.
> Place the rabbit pieces and brown them on all sides for 10 minutes.
> Deglaze with half a glass of white wine and let it evaporate.
> Add the peppers, mix well, season with salt and pepper, sprinkle with the vegetable broth and cook for another 30 minutes.
> After cooking, remove the rabbit from the heat and place the rabbit and peppers on serving plates.
> Sprinkle with the cooking juices and serve.

Tomatoes rabbit

Servings: 4 I Prep time: 15 minutes I Cook time: 1 hour 15 minutes
Nutrition facts per serving: calories: 360; carbs: 7 gr; protein: 34 gr; fat: 11 gr.

Ingredients
✓ 800 gr of rabbit cut into pieces
✓ 8 cherry tomatoes

✓ Almond flour to taste
✓ 200 ml of vegetable broth
✓ 1 garlic clove
✓ ½ glass of white wine
✓ Olive oil, salt and pepper

Directions
> First, peel and wash the onion and then cut it into thin slices.
> Peel and also wash a clove of garlic and then chop it.
> Wash the rabbit thoroughly under running water and then pat it dry with absorbent paper.
> Put a little almond flour on a plate and flour the rabbit pieces well.
> Put a saucepan on the heat source to heat.
> As soon as it is hot enough, add two tablespoons of olive oil.
> Heat the oil and then add the garlic and brown it.
> Add the onions and brown them for 5 minutes.
> Add the rabbit pieces and cook for 10 minutes, turning them often.
> Season with salt and pepper and add a little white wine.
> Add the peeled tomatoes and broth, cover and cook for 50 minutes, stirring occasionally.
> After cooking, remove the rabbit from the heat and let it rest for a few minutes.
> Put the meat on plates, sprinkle with the cooking juices and serve.

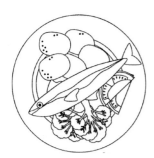

Fish and seafood recipes

Almonds and olives crusted salmon

Servings: 4 I Prep time: 15 minutes I Cook time: 15/20 minutes
Nutrition facts per serving: calories: 420; carbs: 3 gr; protein: 38 gr; fat: 14 gr.

Ingredients
- ✓ 4 salmon fillets of (120 gr for each)
- ✓ 4 thyme sprigs
- ✓ 2 tbsp of chopped almonds
- ✓ 2 tbsp of pitted and chopped black olives
- ✓ Olive oil, salt and pepper

Directions
- ➢ First, clean the salmon fillet.
- ➢ Remove the skin and then wash it very well.
- ➢ Dry salmon fillet with a paper towel.
- ➢ Now you can cut salmon fillets into slices.
- ➢ After that sprinkle them on both sides with salt and pepper.
- ➢ Wash and dry thyme.
- ➢ Place 4 slices of salmon on a cutting board, place 1 thyme sprig inside each slice.
- ➢ Close the slices, sealing them with toothpicks.
- ➢ Mix together the chopped almonds with the chopped black olives.
- ➢ Pass the slices over the almonds and olives breading, pressing them to make the breading adhere well.
- ➢ Heat the olive oil in a pan and as soon as it is hot, put the salmon to brown.
- ➢ Turn them over and cook until the fish is well cooked and golden on the outside.
- ➢ Serve the salmon immediately and hot, sprinkled with the cooking juices.

Aubergine and green pepper trout

Servings: 4 I Prep time: 15 minutes I Cook time: 40 minutes

Nutrition facts per serving: calories: 460; carbs: 6.8 gr; protein:39 gr; fat: 11 gr.

Ingredients
- ✓ 600 gr of trout fillets
- ✓ 1 large aubergine
- ✓ 1 shallot
- ✓ 1 tsp of mint
- ✓ 1 tsp of green pepper grains
- ✓ Olive oil and salt

Directions
- ➢ First, peel the aubergines, wash them, dry them, and then cut them into slices.
- ➢ Put aubergines into a baking pan.
- ➢ Wash and dry mint and then place it in the pan with aubergines.
- ➢ Add one teaspoon of olive oil, salt, and mix.
- ➢ Transfer the pan into preheated oven (180°c).
- ➢ Let cook for 30 minutes about, or until they are well cooked
- ➢ Meanwhile, wash and dry trout filets.
- ➢ Remove the baking pan from the oven and add the trout fillet and the green pepper.
- ➢ Cook for another 10/12 minutes about.
- ➢ When everything will be cooked remove from the oven.
- ➢ Let it rest for a couple of minutes and then cut the trout into slices.
- ➢ Place the aubergines on the bottom of the plate and the trout fillets on top and serve.

Basil and lime mackerel

Servings: 4 I Prep time: 15 minutes I Cook time: 10 minutes
Nutrition facts per serving: calories: 360; carbs: 2 gr; protein: 38 gr; fat: 10 gr.

Ingredients
- ✓ 2 mackerel filets of 250 gram about for each
- ✓ 2 limes juice
- ✓ 1 bunch of fresh parsley, chopped
- ✓ 4 bay leaves
- ✓ Olive oil, salt and pepper in grain

Directions
- ➢ Wash and dry the mackerel fillets.
- ➢ Sprinkle the mackerel fillets with a little salt and pepper and set aside.
- ➢ In a small bowl, put together the lime juice, a tablespoon of olive oil and a pinch of salt and pepper.
- ➢ Combine all ingredients well.
- ➢ Wash parsley leaves, then chop very finely.
- ➢ Take a pan large enough.

➢ Put the mackerel in the pan and brush it with a little olive oil.
➢ Sprinkle the chopped parsley on top.
➢ Put the pan to bake in a preheated oven at 200°c for at least 10 minutes.
➢ Check the cooking and, if necessary, continue cooking for another 5 minutes.
➢ Serve your mackerel dish with cooking juice.

Citrus soy sauce trout

Servings: 4 I Prep time: 60 minutes marnating I Cook time: 20 minutes
Nutrition facts per serving: calories: 420; carbs: 3 gr; protein: 40 gr; fat: 8 gr.

Ingredients
✓ 2 trout fillets of 300 gr about for each
✓ 1 orange
✓ 1 lemon
✓ 1 tsp grated ginger
✓ 1 tbsp of low-carb soy sauce
✓ Olive oil, salt and pepper

Directions
➢ First, take a bowl and mix together the filtered orange and lemon juice, ginger, soy sauce, salt, pepper and a tablespoon of olive oil.
➢ Wash and dry with paper towel the trout fillets and then place them in the bowl with the marinade.
➢ Put to marinate in the fridge for 60 minutes.
➢ After the marinating time, take a pan and place the trout fillets inside.
➢ Sprinkle them with the marinating liquid and then let cook in the oven preheated at 170°c 20 minutes.
➢ As soon as the trout is cooked, remove the pan from the oven.
➢ Place the fish fillets on serving plates and serve immediately sprinkled with the cooking juices.

Cod with red-orange and fennels

Servings: 4 I Prep time: 15 minutes I Cook time: 20 minutes
Nutrition facts per serving: calories: 240; carbs: 5 gr; protein: 30 gr; fat: 1 gr.

Ingredients
✓ 600 gr of cod fillets
✓ 1 red-orange
✓ 1 big fennel

✓ Olive, salt and papper

Directions
➢ Start by cleaning the cod fillets. Wash them under running water, check for bones. In this case, remove them with the help of kitchen tweezers.
➢ Rinse the cod fillets quickly and then dry them with a kitchen towel.
➢ Halve the red-orange, wash it, and cut one half into thin slices.
➢ Wash and dry the internal parts of the fennel.
➢ In a small bowl, mix a tablespoon of oil, half a glass of water, and the orange juice.
➢ Now place the cod fillets in a baking dish or in a pan and season with a pinch of salt and a sprinkling of pepper.
➢ Cover the fish with the orange slices and the fennel.
➢ Pour the orange sauce over the fish.
➢ Cover the ovenproof dish or pan with aluminium foil and place in a preheated oven at 180°c for 15 minutes about.
➢ When it's ready, you can serve your cod dish with fennels and red-orange cooking juice.

Courgette and olives cod

Servings: 4 I Prep time: 10 minutes I Cook time: 20 minutes
Nutrition facts per serving: calories: 310; carbs: 6.8 gr; protein: 29 gr; fat: 6 gr.

Ingredients
✓ 4 cod fillets of 150 gr for each
✓ 2 courgettes
✓ 12 pitted black olives
✓ 1 shallot
✓ ½ bunch of fresh parsley
✓ Olive oil, salt and pepper

Directions
➢ First, peel and wash the courgettes, then cut them into cubes.
➢ Wash and dry the cod fillets and remove all the bones present.
➢ Wash and dry the parsley and chop it.
➢ Peel and wash the shallot and then cut it into thin slices.
➢ Heat two tablespoons of olive oil in a pan and, when it is hot enough, put the parsley and shallots to fry for a few minutes.
➢ Now add the courgettes, mix, season with salt and pepper and continue cooking for 15 minutes.

- ➢ Now add the cod fillets and cook for 8 minutes per side.
- ➢ Now add the black olives, season with salt and pepper, if necessary, leave to flavour for a couple of minutes and turn off.
- ➢ Put the courgettes, cod, and olives on the serving plates.
- ➢ You can serve.

Cucumber fennel seeds and salmon salad

Servings: 4 I Prep time: 1 hour in the feezer + 10 minutes + 10 minutes of marinating I Cook time: -
Nutrition facts per serving: calories: 480; carbs: 2 gr; protein: 49 gr; fat: 10 gr.

Ingredients
- ✓ 600 gr of salmon fillet
- ✓ 4 tbsp of low carb soy sauce
- ✓ 1 tsp of rice vinegar
- ✓ 1 cucumber
- ✓ 2 tsp of fennels seeds
- ✓ Olive oil, salt and pepper

Directions
- ➢ First, place the salmon fillet in the freezer for an hour in order to kill bacteria and make the fillet easier to cut.
- ➢ Meanwhile, prepare salad marinade.
- ➢ In a small bowl, pour the olive oil, soy sauce, rice vinegar, 1 tsp of mixed spices and fennel seeds.
- ➢ After the hour, take the salmon fillet and cut it into strips and put them in a bowl.
- ➢ Pour the marinade over the salmon cubes.
- ➢ Cover everything with cling film and place in the fridge to marinate for 10 minutes.
- ➢ Now, wash the cucumber and cut into thin slices.
- ➢ Now take a bowl and put the salmon cubes.
- ➢ You can also add the cucumber.
- ➢ Sprinkle the salad with a little olive oil salt and pepper. Combine well all ingredients.
- ➢ You can serve the salad.

Dill and orange salmon

Servings: 4 I Prep time: 10 minutes + 20 minutes of marinating I Cook time: -
Nutrition facts per serving: calories: 350; carbs: 2 gr; protein: 30 gr; fat: 7 gr.

Ingredients
- ✓ 4 salmon filets of 100 gr for each
- ✓ 2 oranges

- ✓ 2 tbsp of chopped dill
- ✓ Olive oil, salt and pepper

Directions
- ➢ First, wash the salmon fillets under running water and dry them with paper towels.
- ➢ Wash the oranges thoroughly and then dry them.
- ➢ Divide one of the oranges in half and squeeze it with a juicer.
- ➢ Strain the juice through a fine-mesh strainer.
- ➢ Cut the peel of the squeezed orange into many thin strips.
- ➢ Divide the other orange into many 2 cm thick wedges.
- ➢ Put the salmon fillets with the orange juice in a bowl.
- ➢ Season with salt and pepper, add the chopped dill and cover the salmon.
- ➢ Leave to marinate for at least 20 minutes.
- ➢ Put a plate on the stove and let it heat up.
- ➢ When the plate is hot, place the well-drained salmon fillets.
- ➢ Cook a couple of minutes on each side, but if you prefer more cooking, cook it a few more minutes.
- ➢ Slice the salmon fillets and serve with the orange marinade and some chia seeds sprinkled on top.

Ginger tuna and fennels

Servings: 4 I Prep time: 15 minutes I Cook time: 15 minutes
Nutrition facts per serving: calories: 390; carbs: 3 gr protein: 38 gr fat: 12 gr.

Ingredients
- ✓ 2 tuna fillet (200 gr about for each)
- ✓ 1 tsp of powdered ginger
- ✓ 400 gr of fennels
- ✓ ½ lime
- ✓ Olive oil, salt and pepper

Directions
- ➢ Start with the fennels.
- ➢ Remove the inner part, separate the various leaves, wash them under running water, dry them and then cut the fennel into slices.
- ➢ Also wash some pieces of fennel and set them aside.
- ➢ Take a pan and heat half a tablespoon of oil.
- ➢ Let the oil heat up and then put the fennel slices for about ten minutes to sauté, adding salt and a drop of water.
- ➢ Now switch to the tuna fillet.
- ➢ Wash it under running water. Now take a pan and put 2 sheets of parchment paper inside the pan.

➢ Grease every parchment paper with a little oil. Now add the fish, salt it, sprinkle it with ginger powder and pepper.
➢ Then sprinkle tuna with the lime juice and a drizzle of olive oil and the fennel pieces that you had set aside.
➢ Put the tuna in a preheated oven at 190° c for about 15 minutes.
➢ As soon as they are ready, remove the tuna fillets from the parchment paper, and 4 in four pieces.
➢ Remove the fennel pieces too and place tuna in 4 serving dishes surrounded by previously cooked fennel.
➢ Serve still hot.

Green beans and pistachio salmon

Servings: 4 I Prep time: 10 minutes I Cook time: 20 minutes
Nutrition facts per serving: calories: 450; carbs: 5.8 gr; protein: 41 gr; fat: 10 gr.

Ingredients
✓ 4 salmon fillets of 150 gr for each
✓ 400 gr of green beans
✓ 1 shallot
✓ 4 tbsp of chopped pistachios
✓ Olive oil, salt and pepper

Directions
➢ First, clean the green beans, wash them, and then cut them in half.
➢ Bring a pot of water and salt to a boil and boil the green beans for 5 minutes.
➢ Once cooked, drain, and set aside.
➢ Peel and wash the shallot and then chop it.
➢ Wash and dry the salmon fillets and remove all the bones present.
➢ Wash and dry a bit of parsley and then chop it.
➢ Brush 4 sheets of aluminium foil with oil and then place a salmon fillet in the centre of each sheet.
➢ Put the green beans and shallot inside.
➢ Season with oil, salt and pepper, sprinkle with parsley and chopped pistachios and close the foils.
➢ Place the foils in a baking pan, then transfer the baking pan to the oven and bake at 170°c for 20 minutes.
➢ Once cooked, remove the baking pan from the oven and let it rest for a couple of minutes.
➢ Now put the salmon on the serving plates, surrounded by vegetables and serve.

Green olives and cherry tomatoes cod

Servings: 4 I Prep time: 10 minutes I Cook time: 10/15 minutes
Nutrition facts per serving: calories: 280; carbs: 5 gr; protein: 29 gr; fat: 8 gr.

Ingredients
✓ 4 clean cod filets of 150 gr for each
✓ 12 cherry tomatoes
✓ 2 tbsp of green olives
✓ 1 garlic clove
✓ Olive oil, salt and pepper

Directions
➢ Start by cleaning the cod fillets.
➢ Wash them under tap water, check if there are any bones. In this case, remove them with the help of kitchen tweezers.
➢ Quickly rinse the cod and then dry it with a kitchen towel or parchment paper.
➢ Spread 3 cherry tomatoes cut into fairly small pieces on each sea bass fillet. Add the pitted green olives cut into rings (4 for each cod fillet).
➢ Also cut the garlic into pieces, distributing 1/2 clove on each fish fillet.
➢ Season with salt, add a sprinkling of oregano and sprinkle with a drizzle of olive oil.
➢ Bake the cod in a preheated oven at 190°c for 10-15 minute.
➢ Check the cooking and, if it is ready, you can serve your cod dish still hot.

Mint and almonds prawns

Servings: 4 I Prep time: 10 minutes I Cook time: 10 minutes
Nutrition facts per serving: calories: 280; carbs: 3 gr; protein: 30 gr; fat: 7 gr.

Ingredients
✓ 32 prawns
✓ 2 tbsp of chopped fresh mint
✓ 1 shallot
✓ 4 tbsp of almond flour
✓ 30 ml of almond milk
✓ Olive oil and salt

Directions
➢ First, clean prawns.
➢ Detach the tail and legs from the rest of the body.
➢ Cut the back gently with a knife where the dark filament is.
➢ Remove the filament with the tip of the knife or a toothpick.
➢ Now rinse prawns under running water.

➢ Wash the mint leaves too, and finely chop them with the crescent on a cutting board, together with the peeled shallot.
➢ Now, mix chopped almond, almond milk, chopped mint and shallot, a pinch of pepper, a pinch of salt and the oil in a dish.
➢ Arrange the prawns on a baking sheet and spread a little filling over each one.
➢ Prawns should be well sprinkled.
➢ Grease with a drizzle of oil and bake in a preheated oven at 190°c for about 10 minutes.
➢ At the end of cooking serve mint and almond prawns still hot.

Mustard and coriander sea bass

Servings: 4 I Prep time: 10 minutes + 20 minutes of marinating I Cook time: 15/20 minutes
Nutrition facts per serving: calories: 310; carbs: 6 gr; protein: 29 gr; fat: 4 gr.

Ingredients
✓ 4 sea bass fillets of 150 gr for each
✓ 2 tsp of low-carb soy sauce
✓ 2 little oranges
✓ 1 tbsp of mustard
✓ 1 tbsp of chopped coriander
✓ Olive oil, salt and pepper

Directions
➢ First, wash and dry the coriander, then chop it very finely and transfer to a bowl.
➢ Squeeze both the oranges and take the juice.
➢ Add olive oil, salt, pepper, soy sauce, mustard, and the filtered oranges juice.
➢ Stir and mix everything well.
➢ Wash and dry the sea bass fillets and, if present, remove the bones with tweezers.
➢ Put the fillets in the bowl and marinate them at room temperature for 20 minutes.
➢ Once the marinating time has passed, take a baking pan, and place the sea bass fillets inside.
➢ Sprinkle them with the marinating liquid and let cook at 190°c for 15/20 minutes.
➢ As soon as it is cooked, remove the fish from the oven, place it on serving plates, sprinkle it with the cooking juices and serve.

Orange and parsley tuna

Servings: 4 I Prep time: 10 minutes I Cook time: 15 minutes
Nutrition facts per serving: calories: 360; carbs: 2 gr; protein:38 gr; fat: 10 gr.

Ingredients
✓ 2 tuna fillets of 200 gr about for each
✓ 1 orang, juiced
✓ 1 tbsp of chopped parsley
✓ 1 chopped onion
✓ 1 tbsp of smoked paprika
✓ Olive oil, salt and pepper

Directions
➢ Start the recipe by cleaning the tuna fillets.
➢ Wash them under running water and remove the skin.
➢ Rinse it quickly under running water and then dry it with paper towel.
➢ Sprinkle the fillets with a little salt and pepper and set aside.
➢ In a small bowl, put together the orange juice, a tablespoon of olive oil and chopped onion, a pinch of salt and pepper.
➢ Mix well everything.
➢ Wash parsley, then chop very coarsely.
➢ Take a pan large enough.
➢ Put the tuna in the pan and brush it with a little olive oil.
➢ Sprinkle parsley the on top.
➢ Put the pan to bake in a preheated oven at 180°c for 15 minutes.
➢ Check the cooking and, if necessary, continue cooking for another 5 minutes.
➢ Serve the orange tuna with all the herbs and cooking juice.

Oregano and orange prawns

Servings: 4 I Prep time: 20 minutes of marinating I Cook time: 10 minutes
Nutrition facts per serving: calories: 140; carbs: 2 gr; protein:22 gr; fat: 1 gr.

Ingredients
✓ 24 large prawns
✓ 1 orange juice
✓ 2 tbsp of smoked paprika
✓ 2 tsp of oregano
✓ 1 tbsp of tomato paste
✓ Olive oil, salt and pepper

Directions
➢ First, mix together (in a mixing bowl) olive oil, a bit of coriander, orange juice, smoked paprika, tomato paste, oregano, salt, and black pepper.
➢ A tiny amount should be set aside for basting later
➢ Place the shrimp in a large resalable plastic bag with the remaining marinade. Seal and marinate for 2 hours in the refrigerator.
➢ Preheat the grill to medium-low.

- Thread prawns onto skewers, piercing at the tail and near the head twice.
- Toss out the marinade.
- Lightly grease the grill grate.
- Grill the prawns for 3 minutes per side or until opaque, basting regularly with the marinade you set aside.

Parmesan and pistachio cod

Servings: 4 I Prep time: 10 minutes I Cook time: 20 minutes
Nutrition facts per serving: calories: 380; carbs: 3 gr; protein: 38 gr; fat: 7 gr.

Ingredients
- ✓ 4 cleaned cod fillets of (200 gr for each)
- ✓ 1 onion
- ✓ 2 tbsp rosemary
- ✓ 2 tbsp of chopped pistachios
- ✓ 2 tbsp of grated parmesan cheese
- ✓ Olive oil, salt and pepper

Directions
- Wash and dry cod fillets with a paper towel.
- Cut cod into slices.
- After that sprinkle them on both sides with oil, salt and pepper.
- Place 2 slices of cod on a cutting board.
- Chop onion finely.
- Close the slices with the remaining slices, sealing them with toothpicks.
- Mix together the chopped pistachios with the grated parmesan cheese, onion and rosemary.
- Pass the cod slices over the pistachios and parmesan cheese, pressing them to make the breading adhere well.
- Heat the olive oil in a pan and as soon as it is hot, put the cod to brown.
- Turn them over and cook until the fish is well cooked and golden on the outside.
- Serve the crusted cod immediately and hot, sprinkled with the cooking juices.

Parsley and hazelnut scallops

Servings: 4 I Prep time: 15 minutes I Cook time: 15 minutes
Nutrition facts per serving: calories: 260; carbs: 3 gr; protein: 22 gr; fat: 9 gr.

Ingredients
- ✓ 20 scallops
- ✓ 2 tbsp of chopped parsley
- ✓ 1 garlic clove

- ✓ 50 gr of chopped hazelnuts
- ✓ Olive oil, salt and pepper

Directions
- First, open the scallops.
- Do it, using a knife to force between the two valves, then detach them from the shell, remove the filamentous part and the dark part with the help of kitchen scissors.
- Wash well under fresh running water, very carefully because there are often sand residues.
- Wash the shell well if it is very dirty use a steel wool.
- Peel, wash, and mince garlic clove.
- Wash the parsley too, and finely chop the leaves with.
- Chop the hazelnuts too.
- Chop parsley and mix together with the peeled garlic clove.
- Now, mix chopped hazelnuts, chopped garlic and parsley, a pinch of pepper, a pinch of salt and the oil in a dish.
- Arrange the scallops on a baking sheet and spread a little filling over each one.
- Grease with a drizzle of oil and bake in a preheated oven at 200° c for about 12 minutes.
- At the end of cooking serve the scallops au gratin with hazelnuts and parsley, still hot.

Pecans crusted mackerel

Servings: 4 I Prep time: 1 hour of rest in the fridge + 10 minutes I Cook time: 15/20 minutes
Nutrition facts per serving: calories: 460; carbs: 3 gr; protein: 43 gr; fat: 14 gr.

Ingredients
- ✓ 2 mackerel fillets of 300 gr about for each
- ✓ 1 tsp of smoked paprika
- ✓ 6 tbsp of chopped pecans
- ✓ 3 tbsp of olive oil
- ✓ Salt and pepper to taste

Directions
- Start by putting the mackerel fillet in the freezer for at least an hour.
- After the hour, remove the fish from the freezer, rinse it and dry it with a paper towel.
- Cut it lengthwise to obtain slices.
- Try not to cut too thick slices.
- Put the mackerel slices in a baking tray and sprinkle them with a bit of olive oil.
- Season mackerel slices with smoked paprika, salt and pepper.
- Take the slices of mackerel and pass them in the pecans breading making sure to press well so that it is breaded on all sides.

- ➢ Put a tablespoon of olive oil in a non-stick pan and let it heat up.
- ➢ As soon as the oil starts to sizzle, place the pecans and paprika breaded fish slices in the pan and cook them for a couple of minutes on both sides.
- ➢ Cook until the fish has just turned a lighter pink, or it would be overcooked.
- ➢ As soon as the slices of breaded mackerel are cooked, place it on a serving dish and serve.

Pineapple and lime tuna

Servings: 4 I Prep time: 15 minutes I Cook time: 10 minutes
Nutrition facts per serving: calories: 440; carbs: 8.8 gr; protein: 39 gr; fat: 10 gr.

Ingredients
- ✓ 4 tuna filets of 120 gr for each
- ✓ 300 gr of pineapple pulp
- ✓ 1tsp of rosemary
- ✓ 1 lime zest
- ✓ Olive oil, salt and pepper

Directions
- ➢ Start the recipe by washing the filets of tuna under running water.
- ➢ After washing and rinsing them, drain them and dry them with a kitchen paper towel.
- ➢ Massage tuna fillets with salt and pepper.
- ➢ Add the washed and chopped rosemary.
- ➢ Meanwhile, peel and take the pulp from pineapple.
- ➢ Wash pineapple pulp and cut it into pieces.
- ➢ Mix pineapple pieces with a lime juice. Combine well all ingredients.
- ➢ Cook the tuna at maximum power of your microwave (800 watts) for 3 minutes.
- ➢ When cooking is arrived at 2 minutes, add lime pineapple pieces.
- ➢ If you are not satisfied with the cooking, cook for another minute.
- ➢ When both will be done, you can serve your tuna in serving dishes.

Pistachio chilli tuna

Servings: 4 I Prep time: 1 hour in the freezer (at least) + 10 minutes I Cook time: 15/20 minutes
Nutrition facts per serving: calories: 460; carbs: 3 gr; protein: 43 gr; fat: 14 gr.

Ingredients
- ✓ 4 tuna fillets of 100 gr about

- ✓ 50 gr of chopped pistachios
- ✓ 1 pinch of chilli powder
- ✓ Olive oil, salt and pepper

Directions
- ➢ Start by putting the tuna fillets in the freezer for at least an hour so that as soon as it comes out of the freezer it will be easier to cut it into fillets without breaking the fibres.
- ➢ After the hour, remove the fish from the freezer, rinse it and dry it with a paper towel.
- ➢ Cut it lengthwise to obtain slices.
- ➢ Try not to cut too thick slices.
- ➢ Put the tuna slices in a baking tray and sprinkle them with a little olive oil.
- ➢ Season tuna slices with chilli powder, salt, and pepper.
- ➢ Take the slices of tuna and pass them in the pistachio breading making sure to press well so that it is breaded on all sides.
- ➢ Put a tablespoon of oil in a non-stick pan and let it heat up.
- ➢ As soon as the oil starts to sizzle, place the breaded fish slices in the pan and cook them for a couple of minutes on both sides.
- ➢ Cook until the tuna has just turned a lighter pink, or it would be overcooked.
- ➢ As soon as the slices of breaded tuna with pistachios are cooked, place it on a serving dish and serve.

Porcini mushrooms and tomatoes salmon

Servings: 4 I Prep time: 10 minutes I Cook time: 20 minutes
Nutririon facts: calories: 420; carbs: 6 gr: protein: 40 gr; fat: 12 gr.

Ingredients
- ✓ 4 salmon fillets (120 gr for each), skinless
- ✓ 400 gr of porcini mushrooms
- ✓ 8 cherry tomatoes
- ✓ 1 garlic clove
- ✓ 1 orange
- ✓ Olive oil, salt and pepper

Directions
- ➢ First, preheat the oven to 180°c.
- ➢ Clean salmon fillets under running water and dry them.
- ➢ Clean and dry the porcini mushrooms.
- ➢ Cut mushrooms into 4 pieces.
- ➢ Peel and chop the garlic.
- ➢ Wash cherry tomatoes then halve.
- ➢ Spread some baking paper on a baking sheet.
- ➢ Place the vegetables in the centre of the pan.

- ➤ Place the salmon fillets on the side.
- ➤ Season salmon fillets with salt and pepper.
- ➤ Squeeze the orange over it and drip the olive oil.
- ➤ Close the parchment paper creating a sort of foil.
- ➤ Cook the salmon in a preheated oven for about 20 minutes.
- ➤ Always check the cooking of the salmon and vegetables.
- ➤ You can serve when the salmon and vegetables are cooked.
- ➤ Place salmon surrounded by tomatoes and porcini in serving plates and serve.

Rosemary tuna with courgette and mushrooms

Servings: 4 I Prep time: 10 minutes I Cook time: 20 minutes
Nutrition facts per serving: calories 450; carbs: 6.8 gr; protein:44 gr; fat: 9 gr.

Ingredients
- ✓ 2 tuna fillet (250 gr about for each)
- ✓ 1 courgette
- ✓ 200 gr of mushrooms
- ✓ 1 garlic clove
- ✓ 3 rosemary sprigs
- ✓ Olive oil, salt and pepper

Directions
- ➤ First, preheat the oven to 180°c.
- ➤ Meanwhile, clean the tuna fillet under running water, and dry it.
- ➤ Proceed, in the meantime, washing the courgette.
- ➤ Clean the mushrooms too with a cloth, removing any soil.
- ➤ Cut the courgette into slices and the mushrooms into 4 pieces.
- ➤ Peel and chop the garlic clove too.
- ➤ Spread some baking paper on a baking sheet.
- ➤ Place the vegetables in the centre of the pan.
- ➤ Place the tuna fillet on the side.
- ➤ Season fillets with salt and pepper.
- ➤ Add the rosemary sprig.
- ➤ Close the parchment paper creating a sort of foil.
- ➤ Cook the tuna in a preheated oven for about 20 minutes.
- ➤ Always check the cooking of the fish, courgette, and mushrooms.
- ➤ You can serve when the fish and vegetables are cooked.

Sea bass with asparagus and basil yogurt sauce

Servings: 4 I Prep time: 10 minutes I Cook time: 15 minutes
Nutrition facts per serving: calories: 290; carbs: 7.7 gr; protein: 28 gr; fat: 7 gr.

Ingredients
- ✓ 600 gr of sea bass fillet
- ✓ 400 gr of asparagus
- ✓ 200 ml of greek yogurt
- ✓ 4 basil leaves
- ✓ Olive oil, salt and pepper

Directions
- ➤ First, remove the hardest part from the asparagus. Wash them and then let them drain.
- ➤ Bring a pot of water and salt to a boil and, when it starts to boil, put the asparagus to cook.
- ➤ Cook them for 10 minutes, then drain and let them cool.
- ➤ Wash and dry the sea bass fillet and then remove all the bones present.
- ➤ Cut the fish into four smaller fillets.
- ➤ Wash and dry basil leaves and then chop them.
- ➤ Heat a tablespoon of olive oil in a pan and, when it is hot enough, put the sea bass to cook.
- ➤ Cook for 4 minutes on each side, season with salt and pepper and then turn off.
- ➤ Put the asparagus on the serving plates and place the sea bass on top.
- ➤ Meanwhile prepare the basil yogurt sauce. Put the yogurt, salt, pepper, basil, in a bowl. Mix well until you get a homogeneous mixture.
- ➤ Pour the yogurt sauce over the sea bass and asparagus and then serve.

Spinach and walnuts scallops

Servings: 4 I Prep time: 10 minutes I Cook time: 10/15 minutes
Nutrition facts per serving: calories: 260; carbs: 5 gr; protein: 20 gr; fat: 0 gr; fibre.

Ingredients
- ✓ 16 scallops
- ✓ 200 gr of spinach leaves for salad
- ✓ ½ lemon juice
- ✓ 40 gr of chopped walnuts
- ✓ Olive oil, salt and pepper

Directions
- ➤ First, open the scallops and remove them from their shells.

➤ Use a knife to force between the two valves, then detach them from the shell, remove the filamentous part and the dark part with the help of kitchen scissors.
➤ Wash well under fresh running water. After that, removing them from their shells, rinse and dry them well.
➤ Massage the scallops with salt and pepper to season them.
➤ Now, wash the salad spinach well and drain them.
➤ Heat a pan over medium heat with the olive oil.
➤ Add the scallops and sauté them quickly, 2 minutes per side.
➤ After 4 minutes, remove from heat and set aside.
➤ Put the same pan back on the heat by adding the olive oil again (but this time over high heat) scraping the bottom well with a wooden spoon.
➤ Brown the spinach, stirring for 2-3 minutes until wilted.
➤ Salt and pepper.
➤ Add the chopped walnuts and drizzle with lemon juice.
➤ You can serve by spreading the spinach on a serving plate.
➤ Place the scallops on top of the spinach and serve.

Turmeric tuna and blueberries

Servings: 4 I Prep time: 1 hour in the freezer + 15 minutes for marinating I Cook time: 20 minutes
Nutrition facts per serving: calories: 420; carbs: 9 gr; protein: 39 gr; fat: 8 gr; fibre.

Ingredients
✓ 4 tuna fillets (120 gr about for each)
✓ 2 tbsp of lemon juice
✓ 1 tsp of turmeric powder
✓ 400 gr of blueberries
✓ Olive oil, salt and pepper
Directions
➤ Before starting recipe, let the tuna fillet for at least an hour in the freezer.
➤ After the hour has passed, take it out, rinse and let it dry well.
➤ Start combining, in a small bowl, all the spices.
➤ Mix the oil, turmeric and a bit of salt and pepper well.
➤ Put the tuna in a large bowl and pour the marinade over it.
➤ Leave the fish to marinate for at least 15 minutes in the fridge.
➤ After this time, heat a pan with olive oil.

➤ Take the tuna out of the fridge and cook it directly in the pan with the marinade.
➤ Cook the fish for 3 minutes on the side, taking care not to overcook it.
➤ While the fish is cooking, season the blueberries with the lemon juice.
➤ When the tuna is ready, you can flake it and serve it on serving plates.
➤ Complete the dish, surround tuna fillets with lemon seasoned blueberries.

Vinegar tomatoes and parsley scallops

Servings: 4 I Prep time: 10 minutes I Cook time: 15 minutes
Nutrition facts per serving: calories: 170; carbs: 6 gr; protein:18 gr; fat: 1 gr; fibre.

Ingredients
✓ 24 scallops
✓ 2 tsp of chopped parsley
✓ 12 cherry tomatoes
✓ 1 lime juice
✓ 1 garlic clove
✓ Olive oil, salt and pepper
Directions
➤ Firstly, clean the scallops.
➤ Clean them using a knife to force between the two valves, then detach them from the shell, remove the filamentous part and the dark part with the help of kitchen scissors.
➤ Wash well under fresh running water, very carefully because there are often sand residues.
➤ Wash the shell well if it is very dirty use a steel wool.
➤ Meanwhile wash the parsley tuft and then dry it. Now chop it finely.
➤ Wash the cherry tomatoes, dry them, and halve.
➤ Peel and clean the garlic clove then cut it into thin slices.
➤ Put together 2 tbsp of lime juice, parsley, garlic, salt, pepper in a bowl.
➤ Mix everything well.
➤ Put the scallops in a bowl and cover with the marinade. Put to marinate for 30 minutes in the fridge.
➤ After the time has passed, cut 4 pieces of aluminium large enough to hold 6 scallops per piece.
➤ Put the scallops in the foil, drizzle with a little marinating liquid and sprinkle with the cherry tomatoes. Season with salt and pepper and close the packets.

- ➤ Put the prawns to cook in a preheated oven at 190°c for 10 minutes.
- ➤ Check the cooking, if they are cooked, cook the other packets otherwise continue for another 2 minutes.
- ➤ Serve the scallops hot.

Vinegar tuna with asparagus

Servings: 4 I Prep time: 10 minutes I Cook time: 15 minutes
Nutrition facts per serving: calories: 400; carbs: 3 gr; protein: 38 gr; fat: 7 gr.

Ingredients
- ✓ 4 tuna fillets of 150 gr for each
- ✓ 200 ml of apple cider vinegar
- ✓ 400 gr of green asparagus
- ✓ 2 shallots
- ✓ 1 lemon
- ✓ Olive oil, salt and pepper

Directions
- ➤ First clean asparagus. Remove the final part and the most woody and hard part from the asparagus. Wash and dry them.
- ➤ Brush a baking pan with olive oil and place the asparagus inside, one next to the other.
- ➤ Season them with oil, salt, pepper, and vinegar.
- ➤ Place the baking pan in the oven and bake at 170°c for 5 minutes.
- ➤ In the meantime, remove the skin and all the bones from the tuna fillet, then wash and dry it.
- ➤ Peel and wash the shallot and then cut it into thin slices.
- ➤ Wash and dry the lemon and then cut it into slices.
- ➤ After 5 minutes, remove the baking pan from the oven and place the tuna fillets on top of the asparagus.
- ➤ Season with oil, salt, and pepper, add the slices of shallot, a bit of apple cider vinegar and the lemon slices and put the baking pan back in the oven.
- ➤ Always cook at 170° c for another 25 minutes.
- ➤ Once cooked, remove the baking pan from the oven and let it rest for a couple of minutes.
- ➤ Now put the asparagus and tuna on the serving plates.
- ➤ Decorate with lemon slices and serve.

Walnuts and tofu salmon

Servings: 4 I Prep time: 15 minutes I Cook time: 15/20 minutes
Nutrition facts per serving: calories: 440; carbs: 5 gr; protein: 43 gr; fat: 14 gr.

Ingredients
- ✓ 4 salmon fillets of (120 gr for each)
- ✓ 4 bay leaves
- ✓ 3 tbsp of chopped walnuts
- ✓ 2 tbsp of grated tofu cheese
- ✓ Olive oil, salt and pepper

Directions
- ➤ Start by cleaning the salmon fillet.
- ➤ Remove the skin and then wash it very well.
- ➤ Dry salmon fillet with a paper towel.
- ➤ Now you can cut salmon fillets into slices.
- ➤ After that sprinkle them on both sides with salt and pepper.
- ➤ Wash and dry bay leaves.
- ➤ Place 4 slices of salmon on a cutting board, place 1 bay leaf inside each slice.
- ➤ Close the slices, sealing them with toothpicks.
- ➤ Mix together the chopped walnuts with the grated tofu cheese.
- ➤ Pass the slices over the tofu and walnuts breading, pressing them to make the breading adhere well.
- ➤ Heat the olive oil in a pan and as soon as it is hot, put the salmon to brown.
- ➤ Turn them over and cook until the fish is well cooked and golden on the outside.
- ➤ Serve the salmon immediately and hot, sprinkled with the cooking juices.

Yogurt rocket and avocado prawn salad

Servings: 4 I Prep time: 10 minutes I Cook time: 15 minutes
Nutrition facts per serving: calories: 320; carbs: 5 gr; protein: 30 gr; fat: 15 gr.

Ingredients
- ✓ 800 gr of prawns
- ✓ 1 avocado
- ✓ 120 gr of rocket salad
- ✓ 1 lime
- ✓ 4 tbsp of greek yogurt
- ✓ Olive oil, salt and pepper

Directions
- ➤ You can start with cleaning the prawns. Detach the tail and legs from the rest of the body.
- ➤ Cut the back gently with a knife where the dark filament is.

- ➢ Remove the filament with the tip of the knife or a toothpick.
- ➢ Now rinse prawns under running water.
- ➢ Once cleaned, put the prawns in a bowl and season with salt, pepper, and olive oil.
- ➢ Set the bowl with the prawns aside and let them cook for at least 10 minutes.
- ➢ Now switch to the avocado.
- ➢ Peel and remove the stone inside.
- ➢ Cut half avocado lengthwise to obtain 8 slices.
- ➢ Take a grill and let it heat up.
- ➢ As soon as it is hot enough, take the avocado slices and grill one minute on each side.
- ➢ Set the avocado aside and now switch to grilling the prawns.
- ➢ Let them cook for a couple of minutes on each side. As soon as they are ready, put them on a plate and let them cool.
- ➢ Now move on to preparing the salad. Clean rocket salad under running water and dry it.
- ➢ Put lettuce in a bowl and season them with a mix of oil, salt, and pepper.
- ➢ Set the vegetables aside and go on to prepare the salad dressing sauce.
- ➢ Grate the lime zest and place it in a bowl with the greek yogurt.
- ➢ Then squeeze the lime and add the juice to the bowl.
- ➢ Mix everything well with a spoon.
- ➢ In a serving dish, place the vegetables and avocado on the bottom.
- ➢ Put the prawns on top and finish with the sauce.

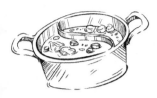

Broth and soups recipes

Avocado lemon and yogurt cold soup

Servings: 4 I Prep time: 10 minutes + 30 minutes of rest in the fridge I Cook time: -
Nutrition facts per serving: calories: 270; carbs: 5 gr; protein: 7 gr; fat: 20 gr.

Ingredients
- ✓ 2 avocados
- ✓ 500 ml of vegetable broth
- ✓ 200 ml of greek yogurt
- ✓ 1 lemon juice
- ✓ Olive oil, salt and pepper

Directions
- ➤ First, peel the avocados, remove the central stones, and then wash them and cut them into cubes.
- ➤ Put the avocado cubes in a bowl and toss with 1 lemon juice.
- ➤ Now pour the greek yogurt into the bowl.
- ➤ Mix gently and then transfer the mixture into the blender.
- ➤ Also add the vegetable broth and blend everything until you get a smooth and homogeneous mixture.
- ➤ Pour the mixture into a tureen, season with salt and pepper, and then let it cool in the refrigerator for 30 minutes.
- ➤ Sprinkle the soup with some chopped chives.
- ➤ You can serve your cold soup.

Basil cucumber cold soup

Servings: 4 I Prep time: 10 minutes + 20 minutes of rst in the fridge I Cook time: -
Nutrition facts per serving: calories: 125; carbs: 5 gr; protein: 7 gr; fat: 6 gr.

Ingredients
- ✓ 4 small cucumbers
- ✓ 1 tbsp of apple cider vinegar
- ✓ 200 ml of vegetable broth
- ✓ 4 basil leaves
- ✓ Olive oil, salt and pepper

Directions

- ➤ First, peel the cucumbers. Wash them and cut one into slices.
- ➤ Cut the others in half and remove the seeds.
- ➤ Cut the cucumbers into chunks and then put them in the glass of the blender. Add the broth, two tablespoons of olive oil, salt, pepper, and 1 tbsp of apple cider vinegar.
- ➤ Blend until smooth and then transfer the soup to the fridge for 20 minutes.
- ➤ Now pour the soup into 4 bowls. Place the cucumber slices on top, sprinkle with the chopped basil leaves and serve.

Chicken ginger broth

Servings: 4 I Prep time: 10 minutes I Cook time: 40 minutes
Nutrition facts per serving: calories: 310; carbs: 2.8 gr; protein: 35 gr; fat: 3 gr.

Ingredients
- ✓ 500 gr of breast chicken chopped into cubes
- ✓ 2 tbsp of grated ginger
- ✓ 2 garlic cloves
- ✓ 600 ml of hot vegetable broth
- ✓ Olive oil, salt and pepper

Directions
- ➤ Peel the garlic cloves and then chop finely.
- ➤ Brown the garlic cloves in a saucepan.
- ➤ As soon as they are golden brown, add ginger and cook for 30 seconds.
- ➤ Now add the chicken and the broth, season with salt and pepper.
- ➤ Cook for 20 minutes, stirring gently.

Chicken and leek soup

Servings: 4 I Prep time: 10 minutes I Cook time: 50 minutes
Nutrition facts per serving: calories: 276; carbs: 6 gr; protein: 21 gr; fat: 10 gr.

Ingredients
- ✓ 400 gr of chicken breast
- ✓ 1 leek
- ✓ 1 shallot
- ✓ 2 bay leaves
- ✓ 1 sprig of thyme
- ✓ Olive oil, salt and pepper

Directions
- ➤ First, wash and dry the chicken breast. Remove the excess fat and then cut it into thin strips.
- ➤ Peel and wash the shallot and then chop it.

- Remove the green party and the outer leaves from the leek. Wash it and then cut it into slices.
- Wash and dry bay leaves and thyme.
- Heat a tbsp of olive oil in a saucepan.
- When it is hot enough, sauté the shallot and leek for 5 minutes.
- Now add the thyme and bay leaf and mix.
- Cook for a couple of minutes and then add the chicken.
- Sauté for 5 minutes and then add 500 ml of water.
- Bring to a boil, season with salt and pepper.
- Lower the heat and continue cooking for another 40 minutes.
- After cooking, turn off and remove the aromatic herbs from the soup.
- Now put the soup on the plates, season it with a drizzle of oil and serve.

Clams and yogurt soup

Servings: 4 I Prep time: 10 minutes I Cook time: 15 minutes
Nutrition facts per serving: calories: 240; carbs: 5 gr; protein: 20 gr; fat: 7 gr.

Ingredients
- ✓ 300 gr of clams
- ✓ 1 shallot
- ✓ 60 gr of greek yogurt
- ✓ 2 sprigs of chopped parsley
- ✓ 1 sprig of thyme
- ✓ Olive oil, salt and pepper

Directions
- Peel and wash the shallot and then cut it into thin slices.
- Scrape the shell of the clams, remove the external beard, and then wash them thoroughly under running water.
- Wash and dry the thyme sprig.
- Put the clams and thyme in a pan, cover them with a lid and let them open.
- As soon as they open, remove them from the pan and remove the shell that does not contain the mollusc. Strain the cooking juices into another bowl.
- Put a tablespoon of olive oil in a saucepan and let it heat up.
- As soon as it is hot, sauté the shallot for a couple of minutes.
- Now add the cooking juices and the yogurt and mix well.
- Cook for 5 minutes and then add the clams.

- Cook for a couple of minutes, season with salt and pepper and then turn off.
- Put the soup on serving plates, sprinkle with chopped parsley and serve.

Coconut and broccoli soup

Servings: 4 I Prep time: 10 minutes I Cook time: 15 minutes
Nutrition facts per serving: calories: 140; carbs: 5.8 gr; protein: 8 gr; fat: 9 gr.

Ingredients
- ✓ 600 gr of broccoli flowers
- ✓ 500 ml of vegetable broth
- ✓ 1 clove of garlic
- ✓ 100 ml of coconut milk
- ✓ 2 tbsp of chopped almonds
- ✓ Olive oil, salt and pepper

Directions
- First, wash the broccoli flowers and then put them to drain.
- Peel the garlic clove.
- Put a little olive oil in a saucepan and put the garlic to brown.
- As soon as it is golden brown, add the broccoli.
- Mix and then add the coconut milk.
- Mix, season with salt and pepper, add a pinch of pepper and then add the vegetable broth.
- When the broccoli is cooked, turn it off and blend everything with an immersion blender.
- Pour the cream into serving dishes.
- Season with olive oil and sprinkle with chopped almonds and, optional: a bit of chopped chives.
- You can serve your soup.

Courgette and cinnamon broth

Servings: 4 I Prep time: 10 minutes I Cook time: 20/30 minutes
Nutrition facts per serving: calories: 100; carbs: 3 gr; protein: 9 gr; fat: 4 gr.

Ingredients
- ✓ 600 gr of courgettes
- ✓ 1 shallot
- ✓ 1 tsp of turmeric
- ✓ 1 tsp of cinnamon
- ✓ 500 ml of hot vegetable broth
- ✓ Olive oil, salt and pepper

Directions

- First, peel the courgettes, wash them, and then cut them into cubes.
- Peel the shallot and chop it finely.
- Brown the shallot pieces in a saucepan.
- As soon as they are golden brown, add all turmeric and cinnamon and cook for 30 seconds.
- Now add the courgettes cubes.
- Mix, season with salt and then add the vegetable broth.
- Cook until the courgettes are very soft.
- At this point turn off and with an immersion blender, blend until you get a thick and velvety cream.
- Put the broth on serving plates, season with a drizzle of oil and the chopped chives and serve.

Mushrooms and oat soup

Servings: 4 I Prep time: 10 minutes I Cook time: 15 minutes
Nutrition facts per serving: calories: 80; carbs: 2 gr; protein: 8 gr; fat: 3 gr.

Ingredients
- ✓ 400 gr of mushrooms
- ✓ 20 gr of grated ginger
- ✓ 300 ml of hot vegetable broth
- ✓ 80 ml of almond milk
- ✓ 1 chilli
- ✓ Olive oil, salt and pepper

Directions
- First, remove any party earth of mushrooms. Clean them well and cut into pieces.
- Put some oil to heat in a pan and then sauté the chilli for a minute.
- Now add the mushrooms and ginger, stir, and cook for 5 minutes.
- Add the vegetable broth and bring to a boil.
- Now add the almond milk and cook until the mushrooms are soft.
- Season with salt and pepper and then turn off.
- Take an immersion blender and blend everything.
- Put the soup on plates, season with oil and pepper and serve.

Mussel courgette and saffron soup

Servings: 4 I Prep time: 10 minutes I Cook time: 20 minutes
Nutrition facts per serving: calories: 230; carbs: 7.8 gr; protein: 20 gr; fat: 5 gr.

Ingredients for servings
- ✓ 300 gr of mussels, cleaned and ready to be cooked
- ✓ 2 medium courgettes
- ✓ 100 gr of peeled tomato
- ✓ 700 ml of vegetable broth
- ✓ 1 garlic glove
- ✓ 1 tsp of saffron
- ✓ Olive oil, salt and pepper

Directions
- Put the mussels in a pan, so that they open.
- As soon as they are all open, turn them off, put them in a bowl and strain the cooking juices into another bowl.
- Wash the courgettes and then cut them into thin slices.
- Peel and wash a garlic clove.
- Heat a tablespoon of oil in a pan and as soon as it is hot, brown the garlic.
- As soon as it is golden brown, remove it and add the courgettes and the peeled tomato.
- Cook for 5 minutes, add the mussels and mix.
- Now add the cooking juices, broth and saffron.
- Stir, season with salt and pepper, and continue cooking for another 10 minutes.
- As soon as the soup is ready, turn it off and immediately put it on serving plates.
- Season with a drop of raw oil and serve.

Pumpkin walnuts and tofu soup

Servings: 4 I Prep time: 10 minutes I Cook time: 10 minutes
Nutrition facts per serving: calories: 210; carbs: 6 gr; protein: 18 gr; fat: 7 gr.

Ingredients
- ✓ 300 gr of pumpkin pulp
- ✓ 1 onion
- ✓ 120 gr of tofu
- ✓ 4 tbsp of chopped walnuts
- ✓ 400 ml of vegetable broth
- ✓ 1 pinch of sweet paprika
- ✓ Olive oil, salt and pepper

Directions
- First, peel the pumpkin and remove the filaments, seeds and take only pulp.
- Wash the pumpkin pulp and then cut it into cubes.
- Peel the onion, wash it, and cut it into slices.
- Put a little oil in a saucepan and when it is hot, put the onion to brown.
- Add now, the pumpkin cubes. Season with salt and pepper and mix well.
- Add a pinch of paprika and mix again.

➢ Now pour the vegetable broth. Cook until all the pumpkin cubes are soft.
➢ In the meantime, rinse the tofu and then pat it under running water.
➢ Heat a grill and when it is hot, grill the tofu for 2-3 minutes per side.
➢ Just cooked, put it on a cutting board and cut into cubes.
➢ Put the tofu in a bowl and season it with a bit of apple cider vinegar.
➢ As soon as the pumpkin and onion are cooked, turn off and blend everything with an immersion blender.
➢ Then put the soup on serving plates, add the tofu cubes, sprinkle with chopped walnuts, and serve.

Spinach in broth

Nutrition facts per serving: calories: 110; carbs: 3 gr; protein: 7 gr; fat: 8 gr.
Servings: 4 I Prep time: 10 minutes I Cook time: 25 minutes

Ingredients
✓ 800 gr of fresh spinach
✓ 1 shallot
✓ 700 ml of hot vegetable broth
✓ 3 tablespoons of cooking vegetable cream
✓ Olive oil, salt and pepper

Directions
➢ Wash and dry the spinach.
➢ Peel the shallot and then cut it into rings.
➢ Put two tablespoons of olive oil in a saucepan.
➢ As soon as it is hot enough, put the shallot to brown for a couple of minutes.
➢ Now add the spinach, season with salt and pepper and sauté for another 2 minutes.
➢ Finally add the vegetable broth and cook for another 20 minutes, covering the pot with a lid.
➢ After 20 minutes, turn off and, with an immersion blender, blend everything until you get a velvety and homogeneous mixture.
➢ Now add the cream and stir until it is completely blended.
➢ Now pour the spinach broth into serving dishes, season with a drizzle of oil and serve.

Squid and courgette soup

Servings: 4 I Prep time: 15 minutes I Cook time: 20 minutes
Nutrition facts per serving: calories: 220; carbs: 4 gr; protein: 19 gr; fat: 8 gr.

Ingredients
✓ 500 gr of cleaned squid
✓ 1 big courgette
✓ 700 ml of vegetable broth
✓ 1 garlic clove
✓ A sprig of parsley
✓ Olive oil, salt and pepper

Directions
➢ First, wash and dry the cleaned squid and then cut them into rings.
➢ Peel, wash and dry the garlic clove.
➢ Put in a pan to brown some oil and as soon as hot add the garlic clove.
➢ As soon as the garlic is golden brown, remove it and brown the squid rings.
➢ Cook for 10 minutes, season with salt and then remove from heat.
➢ Peel the courgette, wash it, dry it, and then cut it into cubes.
➢ Wash and dry the parsley and then chop it.
➢ Put a drizzle of olive oil and fry the courgette with the parsley for a couple of minutes. Season with salt and pepper, and then the vegetable broth.
➢ Cook for 10 minutes and then add the squid rings, cook for a couple of minutes, and then remove from the heat.
➢ Put the soup in 4 serving plates and serve.

Tofu and bell peppers soup

Servings: 4 I Prep time: 10 minutes I Cook time: 15 minutes
Nutrition facts per serving: calories: 210; carbs: 7.9 gr; protein: 20 gr; fat: 3 gr.

Ingredients
✓ 250 ml of soy milk
✓ 130 gr of tofu
✓ 2 yellow (or red) bell peppers
✓ 1 tsp of grated ginger
✓ 400 ml of vegetable broth
✓ Olive oil, salt and pepper

Directions
➢ First, cut the pepper in half. Remove the cap, seeds, and white filaments. Wash them and then cut into thin strips.
➢ Take a saucepan and heat the bell pepper strips. Broth together with the ginger.
➢ While the broth is heating up, dab the tofu with a paper towel and then cut it into cubes.
➢ Sauté the tofu in a pan with a drizzle of olive oil and a bit of soy sauce for 2-3 minutes, then turn off and set aside.
➢ As soon as the broth comes to a boil, we put

the bell peppers inside.
- ➢ Boil for 2 minutes and then add the soy milk.
- ➢ Mix well and after a couple of minutes add the tofu.
- ➢ Cook for another 5 minutes, season with salt, then turn off.
- ➢ Put the soup on serving plates and serve hot.

Tofu and sesame broth

Servings: 4 I Prep time: 10 minutes I Cook time: 15 minutes
Nutrition facts per serving: calories: 210; carbs: 2 gr; protein: 29 gr; fat: 4 gr.

Ingredients
- ✓ 200 gr of tofu
- ✓ 1 garlic clove
- ✓ 1 tbsp of sesame seeds
- ✓ 2 tbsp of vegan broth
- ✓ 2 tsp of low-carb of soy sauce
- ✓ Olive oil, salt and pepper

Directions
- ➢ First, carefully rinse the tofu, pat it dry with a paper towel then put it in a saucepan covered with cold water and broth.
- ➢ Bring it to a boil, then turn off or lower the heat and keep it warm until ready to serve.
- ➢ In the meantime, prepare the sauce.
- ➢ Peel and wash the garlic and then chop it.
- ➢ Take a bowl and put the minced garlic inside.
- ➢ Add the olive oil (2 tbsp), the soy sauce, the pepper and mix well.
- ➢ Add the sesame seeds and mix again.
- ➢ When the sauce is ready, drain the tofu and pat it with a paper towel.
- ➢ Cut it into slices, put it on plates and sprinkle it with the sauce.
- ➢ Serve immediately while still hot.

Turkey garlic and courgette soup

Servings: 4 I Prep time: 10 minutes I Cook time: 45/50 minutes
Nutrition facts per serving: calories: 290; carbs: 7.7 gr; protein: 21 gr; fat: 10 gr.

Ingredients
- ✓ 400 gr of turkey breast
- ✓ 2 courgettes
- ✓ 1 garlic
- ✓ 1 sprig of rosemary
- ✓ 1 tbsp of powdered ginger
- ✓ Olive oil, salt and pepper

Directions
- ➢ First, wash and dry the turkey breast, removing any excess fat.
- ➢ After that, you can cut it into thin cubes.
- ➢ Wash the courgettes and cut into cubes.
- ➢ Peel and wash the garlic and then chop it.
- ➢ Wash and dry rosemary sprig.
- ➢ Heat a tbsp of olive oil in a saucepan.
- ➢ When it is hot enough, sauté the garlic and courgettes for 5 minutes.
- ➢ Cook for a couple of minutes and then add the turkey cubes.
- ➢ Sauté for 5 minutes and then add 500 ml of water.
- ➢ Bring to a boil, season with salt and pepper and ginger powder.
- ➢ Lower the heat and continue cooking for another 40 minutes.
- ➢ After cooking, turn off and remove the rosemary from the soup.
- ➢ Now put the soup on the plates, season it with a drizzle of oil and serve.

Side dishes

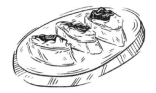

Almonds and grapefruit salad

Servings: 4 I Prep time: 10 minutes I Cook time: -
Nutrition facts *per serving*: calories: 140; carbs: 6.8 gr; protein: 2.8 gr; fat: 6 gr.

Ingredients
- ✓ 1 grapefruit (around 200 gr)
- ✓ 60 gr of chopped almonds
- ✓ 2 chopped parsley leaves
- ✓ 1 chilli
- ✓ 2 tbsp of vinegar

Directions
- ➢ Peel the grapefruit and then cut it into wedges.
- ➢ Wash the chilli, cut it in half, remove the seeds and then cut it into small pieces.
- ➢ Peel and wash the carrot and then cut it into thin slices.
- ➢ Take a salad bowl and put the grapefruit and chilli inside.
- ➢ In a bowl put the vinegar, oil, salt, pepper, and the chopped parsley leaves. Mix well with a fork.
- ➢ Pour the emulsion into the salad bowl and mix everything gently.
- ➢ Sprinkle the salad with chopped almonds and serve.

Basil and garlic baked tomatoes

Servings: 4 I Prep time: 10 minutes I Cook time: 30 minutes
Nutrition facts *per serving*: calories: 90; carbs: 8.7 gr; protein: 1 gr; fat: 3 gr.

Ingredients
- ✓ 500 gr of cherry tomatoes
- ✓ 1 garlic
- ✓ 100 ml of apple cider vinegar
- ✓ A teaspoon of dried oregano
- ✓ 6 chopped basil leaves
- ✓ Olive oil, salt and pepper

Directions
- ➢ Wash the tomatoes and leave them whole.

- ➢ Peel and wash the garlic and then cut its cloves into pieces.
- ➢ Take a baking sheet and brush it with a little oil.
- ➢ Put the cherry tomatoes and the garlic pieces inside.
- ➢ Season with oil, salt, oregano, basil, pepper, and mix to flavour well.
- ➢ Put the pan in the oven and cook at 200 ° for 30 minutes.
- ➢ After the cook time, remove from the oven, put on serving plates and serve.

Beetroot parsley and orange salad

Servings: 4 I Prep time: 10 minutes I Cook time: -
Nutrition facts *per serving*: calories: 80; carbs: 6.8 gr; protein: 2 gr; fat: 3 gr.

Ingredients
- ✓ 1 medium beetroot already cooked
- ✓ 2 blood oranges
- ✓ 1 tbsp of chopped parsley
- ✓ 2 tbsp of apple cider vinegar
- ✓ Olive oil, salt and pepper

Directions
- ➢ First, peel the oranges, then wash and cut them into slices.
- ➢ Peel the cooked beetroot. Cut it into thin slices.
- ➢ Arrange the beetroot slices in a circle on a plate, alternating them with the orange slices.
- ➢ Wash the parsley leaves and chop a tbsp of them.
- ➢ In a bowl put together the chopped parsley, oil, apple cider vinegar, salt and pepper and mix well.
- ➢ Sprinkle blood oranges and beetroot with the vinaigrette and serve.

Coriander grilled aubergine

Servings: 4 I Prep time: 10 minutes I Cook time: 10 minutes
Nutrition facts *per serving*: calories: 170; carbs: 8.7 gr; protein: 4 gr; fat: 6 gr.

Ingredients
- ✓ 2 aubergines
- ✓ 1 tsp of low-carb soy sauce
- ✓ 10 coriander leaves
- ✓ Olive oil, salt and pepper

Directions
- ➢ First wash and trim the aubergines, then cut them into thin slices and set aside.
- ➢ Cut them in 2 parts.

- ➢ Brush the aubergine slices with a little olive oil. Sprinkle with salt and pepper.
- ➢ Heat up a grill and when it is hot, grill the aubergine 3-4 minutes per side.
- ➢ When they are ready put them on a sheet of paper towel and leave them to rest.
- ➢ Wash and dry the coriander leaves.
- ➢ Put them in the glass of the mixer together with a tbsp of olive oil and the soy sauce.
- ➢ Chop everything very finely.
- ➢ On a serving dish lay the slices of aubergine, spread the sauce on the surface of the dish and serve.

Cinnamon braised cucumber

Servings: 4 I Prep time: 10 minutes I Cook time: 50 minutes
Nutrition facts per serving: calories: 50; carbs: 5 gr; protein: 3 gr; fat: 2 gr.

Ingredients
- ✓ 2 big cucumbers
- ✓ 1 stick of celery
- ✓ 1 sprig of rosemary
- ✓ 1 tsp of chopped onion
- ✓ 1 tbsp of ground cinnamon
- ✓ Olive oil, salt and pepper

Directions
- ➢ Peel and wash the cucumbers and then cut it into small pieces.
- ➢ Remove the celery stalk and then wash it and cut it into pieces.
- ➢ Wash the rosemary and take only the needles.
- ➢ Peel, wash, and chop 1 tsp of onion.
- ➢ Put a little oil in a saucepan, and when it is hot, brown the onion, together with the rosemary for a couple of minutes.
- ➢ Now add the celery and cucumber. Season with salt and pepper and then add half a glass of hot water.
- ➢ Cover with a lid and cook for 45 minutes, stirring occasionally.
- ➢ After cook time, remove the lid and sprinkle with cinnamon.
- ➢ Mix, put on serving plates and serve your side dish.

Courgette and rosemary stuffed tomatoes

Servings: 4 I Prep time: 15 minutes I Cook time: 30 minutes

Nutrition facts per serving: calories: 115; carbs: 6.4 gr; protein: 3 gr; fat: 1 gr.

Ingredients
- ✓ 4 big tomatoes of about 100 gr each ones
- ✓ 1 courgette
- ✓ 1 tsp of rosemary
- ✓ Olive oil, salt and pepper

Directions
- ➢ First, wash the tomatoes, cut off the top and with a teaspoon.
- ➢ Remove all seeds.
- ➢ Let them drain upside down and in the meantime move on to preparing the filling.
- ➢ Wash and chop very coarsely rosemary.
- ➢ Peel and cut the courgette into very small pieces.
- ➢ Sauté them in a non-stick pan with a drizzle of oil and a glass of water for about ten minutes, adding the chopped rosemary and salt.
- ➢ Fill the tomatoes with the courgettes, using a teaspoon.
- ➢ Leave them to flavour in the fridge for at least 30 minutes.
- ➢ You can serve.

Creamy yogurt and mustard beets

Servings: 4 I Prep time: 10 minutes I Cook time: 10 minutes
Nutrition facts per serving: calories: 160; carbs: 8.7 gr; protein: 9 gr; fat: 5 gr.

Ingredients
- ✓ 700 gr of beets
- ✓ 150 ml of greek yogurt
- ✓ 1 tbsp of grain mustard
- ✓ 1 tsp of powdered ginger
- ✓ A pinch of nutmeg
- ✓ Olive oil, salt and pepper

Directions
- ➢ Wash the beets under running water.
- ➢ Bring a pot of water and salt to the boil and cook the beets for 3 minutes.
- ➢ Drain them and keep them temporarily aside.
- ➢ Put to heat a little oil in a pan. As soon as it is hot, add the mustard grains, nutmeg, and ginger.
- ➢ When the mustard seeds start to crackle, add the beets.
- ➢ Mix, season with salt, pepper, and leave to flavour for a couple of minutes.
- ➢ Now add the greek yogurt, mix well and let it cook for another minute.
- ➢ Turn off, transfer the mixture to a serving dish and serve your beets dish.

Cucumber and pomegranate salad

Servings: 4 I Prep time: 10 minutes I Cook time: -
Nutrition facts per serving: calories: 90; carbs: 6 gr; protein:4 gr; fat: 5 gr.

Ingredients
- ✓ 1 big cucumber
- ✓ 1 lime
- ✓ 1 pomegranate
- ✓ 30 ml of apple cider vinegar
- ✓ 1 tsp of chia seeds
- ✓ Olive oil, salt and pepper

Directions
- ➤ First, peel, and wash cucumber. Now cut it into thin slices.
- ➤ Wash the lime and then peel it. Cut it into wedges.
- ➤ Cut the pomegranate in half, peel it, and shell the grains.
- ➤ Put lime, pomegranate, and cucumber in a salad bowl.
- ➤ In a small bowl mix together apple cider vinegar, oil, salt, and pepper.
- ➤ Pour the emulsion obtained into the bowl with the vegetables.
- ➤ Mix everything gently, sprinkle with chia seeds and serve your salad.

Cucumber onion and radicchio salad

Servings: 4 I Prep time: 10 minutes I Cook time: -
Nutrition facts per serving: calories: 150; carbs: 7.2 gr; protein: 4 gr; fat: 4 gr.

Ingredients
- ✓ 2 small cucumbers
- ✓ 400 gr of radicchio leaves
- ✓ 1 red onion
- ✓ 1 teaspoon of dried oregano

Directions
- ➤ Wash and dry the radicchio leaves well and then cut them into thin slices.
- ➤ Wash the cucumbers and then cut into slices.
- ➤ Peel and wash the onion and then cut it into slices.
- ➤ Put the radicchio leaves and cucumbers at the bottom of a salad bowl.
- ➤ Now add the onion slice.
- ➤ Season with oil, salt, and pepper.
- ➤ Stir to flavour well, sprinkle with oregano and serve your salad.

Curry lime aubergine

Servings: 4 I Prep time: 10 minutes I Cook time: 20 minutes
Nutrition facts per serving: calories: 190; carbs: 7.2 gr; protein: 3 gr; fat: 7 gr.

Ingredients
- ✓ 1 aubergine (400 gr about)
- ✓ 1 tsp of turmeric
- ✓ 1 tsp of curry
- ✓ 1 shallot
- ✓ 100 ml of unsweetened lime juice

Directions
- ➤ First, peel the aubergines, wash them carefully and then cut them into cubes.
- ➤ Peel and wash the shallot and then chop it.
- ➤ Put the aubergine and shallot in a bowl.
- ➤ Add the turmeric and curry, salt and pepper and mix well.
- ➤ Now put everything in a saucepan and cover the aubergine completely with cold water.
- ➤ Boil the water and continue cooking for another 10 minutes.
- ➤ Now add the lime juice and continue to cook for another 8 minutes.
- ➤ After cooking, turn off and transfer the aubergine to serving plates.
- ➤ Sprinkle with the cooking juices and serve.

Green beans shallot and hazelnuts salad

Servings: 4 I Prep time: 10 minutes I Cook time: 10 minutes
Nutrition facts per serving: calories: 140; carbs: 6.8 gr; protein: 6 gr; fat: 9 gr.

Ingredients
- ✓ 400 gr of green beans
- ✓ 1 shallot
- ✓ 4 tbsp of chopped hazelnuts
- ✓ 30 ml of mustard
- ✓ 1 orange
- ✓ Olive oil, salt and pepper

Directions
- ➤ First, start with cleaning green beans. Remove the end of the green beans and then wash them.
- ➤ Cut the green beans into two parts and then put them to cook in salted boiling water for 10 minutes.
- ➤ Once cooked, drain, and let them cool.
- ➤ Meanwhile, peel and wash the shallot and then cut it into thin slices.

➤ Put the mustard, 1 tbsp of oil, salt, pepper, and the filtered orange juice in a bowl. Stir until you get a homogeneous emulsion.

➤ As soon as the green beans have cooled, put them in a salad bowl.

➤ Add the cherry tomatoes and sprinkle them with the mustard sauce.

➤ Stir to flavour the vegetables well, sprinkle the salad with chopped hazelnuts and serve.

Herbs and walnuts pumpkin

Servings: 4 I Prep time: 10 minutes I Cook time: 40 minutes
Nutrition facts per serving: calories: 220; carbs: 6 gr; protein: 3 gr; fat: 10 gr.

Ingredients
- ✓ 500 gr of pumpkin pulp
- ✓ 2 tbsp of chopped walnuts
- ✓ 1 sprig of thyme
- ✓ 1 sprig of chopped parsley
- ✓ 2 sage leaves
- ✓ Olive oil, salt and pepper

Directions
➤ First, wash the pumpkin pulp and then cut it into slices. Season it with salt and pepper.

➤ Wash and dry the sage and thyme and then chop them.

➤ Brush a baking pan with oil and then put the pumpkin inside.

➤ Sprinkle with a little oil and then sprinkle it with the chopped aromatic herbs, a pinch of paprika and chopped walnuts.

➤ Place the baking pan in the oven and bake at 160°c for 40 minutes.

➤ Once cooked, remove the baking pan from the oven and let the pumpkin rest for a couple of minutes.

➤ Now put the pumpkin on the serving dishes and serve.

Orange and nuts cauliflower

Servings: 4 I Prep time: 10 minutes I Cook time: 15 minutes
Nutrition facts per serving: calories: 120; carbs: 3 gr; protein: 11 gr; fat: 4 gr.

Ingredients
- ✓ 1 cauliflower
- ✓ ½ orange
- ✓ 3 tbsp of chopped hazelnuts
- ✓ 1 tbsp of peeled almonds

- ✓ 2 tbsp of low-carb soy sauce
- ✓ Olive oil, salt and pepper

Directions
➤ First, clean and take only flowers from cauliflower.

➤ Wash them and then cook them in salted boiling water for 12 minutes.

➤ Drain the vegetables and set them aside to cool.

➤ Peel the orange, wash it, and then cut it into wedges.

➤ Put the orange wedges in a bowl together with the cauliflower.

➤ Season with salt, pepper, and a tbsp of olive oil.

➤ Now toast the almonds and hazelnuts in a pan for a couple of minutes.

➤ Put them in the bowl with the rest of the ingredients.

➤ Season with the soy sauce and combine well all ingredients.

➤ Serve your side dish.

Pepper olives and cucumber salad

Servings: 4 I Prep time: 10 minutes I Cook time: 15 minutes
Nutrition facts per serving: calories: 150; carbs: 6.8 gr; protein: 5 gr; fat: 9 gr.

Ingredients
- ✓ 1 big yellow bell pepper
- ✓ 1 big cucumber
- ✓ 10 green olives
- ✓ 3 tbsp of apple cider vinegar
- ✓ 2 tbsp of mustard
- ✓ Olive oil, salt and pepper

Directions
➤ First, wash the yellow pepper. Brush a baking pan with olive oil and put the pepper inside.

➤ Bake in the oven at 200° c for at least 15 minutes.

➤ After cooking, remove the pepper from the oven. Remove the top cap, seeds, and white filaments. Cut it into slices and put it in a bowl to cool.

➤ Meanwhile, wash the cucumber and then cut it into slices.

➤ As soon as the pepper has cooled, put it in a salad bowl.

➤ Add the cucumber and olives.

➤ Add the mustard, vinegar, oil, salt, and pepper to the liquid of the pepper and mix everything well.

➤ Sprinkle the vegetables with the mustard sauce.

➤ Mix well to flavour all the ingredients and serve your salad.

Pineapple and fennel salad

Servings: 4 I Prep time: 10 minutes I Cook time: -
Nutrition facts per serving: calories: 80; carbs: 5 gr; protein: 4 gr; fat: 5 gr.

Ingredients
- ✓ 1 fennel
- ✓ 1 orange
- ✓ ½ pineapple pulp
- ✓ 2 tbsp of apple cider vinegar
- ✓ Olive oil, salt and pepper

Directions
- ➢ First, clean the fennel. Cut the tops and the base, taking care to deprive them of the outer leaves. Wash the fennel under running water, and then dry them. Now cut them into thin slices.
- ➢ Wash the orange and then peel it. Cut it into wedges.
- ➢ Cut the pineapple in half, peel it, and remove the pulp.
- ➢ Wash the pulp and cut into cubes.
- ➢ Put orange, pineapple, and fennel in a salad bowl.
- ➢ In a small bowl mix together vinegar, oil, salt, and pepper.
- ➢ Pour the emulsion obtained into the bowl with the vegetables.
- ➢ Mix everything gently and serve your side dish.

Pistachio and parmesan stuffed courgette

Servings: 4 I Prep time: 10 minutes I Cook time: 45 minutes
Nutrition facts per serving: calories: 190; carbs: 6.9 gr; protein: 14 gr; fat: 7 gr.

Ingredients
- ✓ 2 courgettes
- ✓ 1 small onion
- ✓ 50 gr of chopped pistachios
- ✓ 4 tbsp of grated parmesan cheese
- ✓ 1 sprig of chopped parsley
- ✓ Olive oil, salt and pepper

Directions
- ➢ First, wash and dry the courgettes.
- ➢ Cut them in half lengthwise.
- ➢ With a sharp knife, remove the pulp of the courgettes and cut it into cubes.
- ➢ Peel and wash the onion and then chop it.
- ➢ Heat a tbsp of olive oil in a pan and brown the onion.
- ➢ Add the courgettes pulp, mix, and cook for 4 minutes.
- ➢ Add the pistachio, salt, and pepper, mix, and continue cooking for another 3 minutes.
- ➢ After 3 minutes, turn off and let the mixture cool.
- ➢ As soon as it has cooled, add a mixture of parmesan and parsley.
- ➢ Stir until everything is well incorporated.
- ➢ Take a baking pan and line it with parchment paper.
- ➢ Place the courgettes inside and season with salt and pepper.
- ➢ Now put the filling inside the courgettes.
- ➢ Transfer the baking pan to the oven and bake at 160° c for 30 minutes.
- ➢ After 30 minutes, remove the baking pan from the oven.
- ➢ Let the courgettes rest for 5 minutes, then put them on serving plates and serve.

Red bell peppers in basil sauce

Servings: 4 I Prep time: 10 minutes I Cook time: 10 minutes
Nutrition facts per serving: calories: 160; carbs: 6.8 gr; protein: 2 gr; fat: 7 gr.

Ingredients
- ✓ 2 red bell peppers
- ✓ 1 red onion
- ✓ 1 tbsp of chopped basil
- ✓ 4 tbsp of apple cider vinegar
- ✓ Olive oil, salt and pepper

Directions
- ➢ First, remove the cap from the peppers.
- ➢ Cut them into 4 parts and remove the seeds and white filaments.
- ➢ Wash and dry the peppers and cut the 4 parts into 2.
- ➢ Brush the peppers with olive oil and then season with salt and pepper.
- ➢ Heat a grill and as soon as it is hot, grill the peppers.
- ➢ Cook the peppers for 4 minutes per side.
- ➢ Once cooked, remove them from the grill and place them on a serving dish.
- ➢ Peel and wash the red onion and then cut it into slices.
- ➢ Sprinkle the peppers with the onion and chopped basil.
- ➢ In a bowl, emulsify the vinegar, a tbsp of oil, salt, and pepper together.
- ➢ Sprinkle the red bell peppers with the emulsion and serve.

Rocket walnuts and tomatoes salad

Servings: 4 I Prep time: 10 minutes I Cook time: -
Nutrition facts per serving: calories: 100; carbs: 7.6 gr; protein: 4 gr; fat: 8 gr.

Ingredients for 2 servings
- ✓ 10 cherry tomatoes
- ✓ 300 gr of rocket
- ✓ 6 tbsp of chopped walnuts
- ✓ 2 tbsp of apple cider vinegar
- ✓ Olive oil, salt and pepper

Directions
- ➢ Wash and dry cherry tomatoes, then put on a bowl.
- ➢ Wash and dry the rocket and then put it on top of the tomatoes.
- ➢ Put the oil, salt, pepper, and apple cider vinegar in a bowl and mix well.
- ➢ Sprinkle the rocket and tomatoes with the emulsion.
- ➢ Sprinkle with the chopped walnuts and serve.

Sage and mustard carrot

Servings: 4 I Prep time: 10 minutes I Cook time: 40 minutes
Nutrition facts per serving: calories: 70; carbs: 6.2 gr; protein: 2 gr; fat: 3 gr.

Ingredients
- ✓ 200 gr of carrots
- ✓ 1 teaspoon of grain mustard
- ✓ 1 teaspoon of apple cider vinegar
- ✓ 1 tbsp of chopped sage
- ✓ 1 garlic clove

Directions
- ➢ First, peel and wash the carrots thoroughly and then dry them with a paper towel.
- ➢ Now cut the carrots into four parts, lengthwise.
- ➢ In a bowl, mix mustard grains, apple cider vinegar and a tablespoon of olive oil.
- ➢ Wash and dry the thyme and remove only the leaves.
- ➢ Take a baking sheet and brush it with olive oil.
- ➢ Place the carrots inside and sprinkle them with salt and pepper.
- ➢ Sprinkle with the emulsion and thyme leaves and then bake in the oven at 200 ° c for 35 minutes.
- ➢ After the cook time, take them out of the oven, transfer them to serving dishes and serve.

Walnuts sautéed spinach

Servings: 4 I Prep time: 10 minutes I Cook time: 15 minutes
Nutrition facts per serving: calories: 90; carbs: 4 gr; protein: 8 gr; fat: 5 gr.

Ingredients
- ✓ 800 gr of spinach
- ✓ 4 tsp of chopped walnuts
- ✓ 1 sprig of chopped coriander
- ✓ Olive oil, salt and pepper

Directions
- ➢ First, wash the spinach under running water.
- ➢ Put the spinach in a pan and cook without adding oil or water.
- ➢ Cook for about ten minutes, then turn off and drain.
- ➢ Heat up a little oil in a pan and as soon as it is hot, add the spinach.
- ➢ Add the chopped coriander, season with salt and pepper and mix well.
- ➢ Add the chopped walnuts, cook for another five minutes, and turn off.
- ➢ Put spinach on serving dishes and serve.

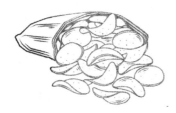

Snack recipes

Almond and chia seeds pudding

Servings: 4 I Prep time: 10 minutes I Cook time: 2 minutes
Nutrition facts per serving: calories: 140; carbs: 5 gr; protein: 10; gr fat: 8 gr.

Ingredients
- ✓ 100 gr of almond flour
- ✓ 70 ml of water
- ✓ 2 tbsp of almond milk
- ✓ 15 gr of greek yogurt
- ✓ 10 gr of chia seeds
- ✓ Olive oil, salt and pepper

Directions
- ➢ First, combine greek yogurt with almond flour, water, almond milk, and chia seeds in a microwave-safe bowl.
- ➢ Microwave for 45 seconds.
- ➢ Then add maple syrup and microwave another 30 seconds.
- ➢ Add additional almond milk if necessary.
- ➢ You can serve your almond pudding still hot.

Almond soy and cucumbers cups

Servings: 4 I Prep time: 10 minutes I Cook time: 45 minutes
Nutrition facts per serving: calories: 120; carbs: 4 gr; protein: 10 gr; fat: 7 gr.

Ingredients
- ✓ 2 cucumbers
- ✓ 800 ml of soy milk
- ✓ 1 tbsp of powdered stevia
- ✓ 80 gr of almonds
- ✓ 1 tbsp of cinnamon powder
- ✓ Olive oil, salt and pepper

Directions
- ➢ First, scrape the cucumbers, wash them, and reduce them to cream with a vegetable mill or blender.
- ➢ Pour the soy milk into a saucepan, add the cucumbers and boil over low heat for about 20 minutes.

- ➢ After the indicated time, add the stevia, mix well and cook over low heat for another 15 minutes.
- ➢ In the meantime, blanch the almonds for a few moments, so as to be able to peel them more easily, blend them and add them to the cucumbers.
- ➢ Add the cinnamon powder too.
- ➢ After the set time, pass the mixture again in the vegetable mill or in the blender, then transfer the cream obtained into individual cups.
- ➢ Keep them cool for at least 30 minutes before serving.
- ➢ You can serve your cups.

Almond courgette and parmesan croquettes

Servings: 4 I Prep time: 10 minutes I Cook time: 45 minutes
Nutrition facts per serving: calories: 250; carbs: 5.8 gr; protein: 15 gr fat: 12 gr.

Ingredients
- ✓ 2 medium courgettes
- ✓ 120 gr of almond flour
- ✓ 2 tbsp of grated parmesan cheese
- ✓ 80 gr of almond flour
- ✓ 50 ml of soymilk cooking cream

Directions
- ➢ First wash and peel courgettes, then cut them into cubes.
- ➢ Boil the courgettes cubes in salted water for 15 minutes.
- ➢ When they will be done, drain and mash finely in a large bowl using a courgettes masher or ricer.
- ➢ Cool completely.
- ➢ Mix with a tbsp of almond milk, parmesan cheese, almond flour in a bowl.
- ➢ Season with a little oil, salt and pepper.
- ➢ Shape the courgettes filling into the size of golf balls and set aside.
- ➢ Preheat the oven to 190°c.
- ➢ Mix the almonds and almond flour and stir until the mixture becomes loose and crumbly. Place each courgettes ball into the soymilk cream and then the almond flour and roll into a croquette shape.
- ➢ Press coating to croquettes to ensure it adheres.
- ➢ Place the croquettes into the baking pan then put it in the oven at 190°c.
- ➢ Let the croquettes cook for 20 minutes or until they become golden brown.
- ➢ Serve hot with a low-carb sauce.

Avocado and oat chips

Servings: 4 I Prep time: 10 minutes I Cook time: 15/20 minutes
Nutrition facts per serving: calories: 180; carbs: 5 gr; protein: 10 gr; fat: 8 gr.

Ingredients
- ✓ 1 avocado
- ✓ 50 gr of oat flour
- ✓ 70 ml water
- ✓ 40 gr of wholemeal breadcrumbs
- ✓ Salt and pepper to taste
- ✓ Olive oil, salt and pepper

Directions
- ➢ First, halve the avocado.
- ➢ Remove the central stone and with the help of a spoon remove the peel.
- ➢ Cut the avocado into slices that are not too thin. In a bowl, dissolve the oat flour with the water, mixing well with a whisk to remove all possible lumps.
- ➢ Season with salt and pepper. In a second bowl pour the breadcrumbs instead.
- ➢ Pass the avocado slices first in the oat flour batter, then in the breadcrumbs and arrange them on a baking sheet lined with parchment paper.
- ➢ Once all the avocado slices have been breaded, bake them in a static oven at 160° c for 15/20 minutes, seasoning them first with a drop of oil to make them golden.
- ➢ Once ready, serve hot or at most lukewarm.

Avocado coconut and orange salad

Servings: 4 I Prep time: 5 minutes + 30 minutes in the fridge I Cook time: -
Nutrition facts per serving: calories: 140; carbs: 4 gr; protein: 8 gr; fat: 10 gr.

Ingredients
- ✓ 1 orange
- ✓ 1 avocado
- ✓ 4 tbsp of coconut flour
- ✓ 40 ml of coconut milk

Directions
- ➢ First, wash and dry the orange. After having wash, it grate the zest and divide the pulp into slices.
- ➢ Peel and wash the avocado too, then halve.
- ➢ Now remove the central stone and cut it into cubes.
- ➢ Put the avocado and oranges in a bowl.
- ➢ Sprinkle the fruit with the coconut milk.
- ➢ Mix gently and then transfer to the fridge for 30 minutes.
- ➢ After 30 minutes, put the fruit salad in two bowls, cover them with the grated orange rind and coconut flour and serve.

Artichokes and cheddar omelette

Nutrition facts per serving: calories: 140; carbs: 5 gr; protein: 11 gr; fat: 6 gr.

Ingredients
- ✓ 6 eggs
- ✓ 250 gr of artichoke hearts
- ✓ 1 tsp of smoked paprika
- ✓ 40 gr of grated cheddar cheese
- ✓ 1 tsp of chopped parsley
  - ✓ Olive oil, salt and pepper

Directions
- ➢ Start with the artichoke hearts.
- ➢ Remove the earthy part, wash them, dry them, and cut them into thin slices.
- ➢ Put the eggs in a bowl and beat them vigorously with a fork.
- ➢ Add a pinch of salt and smoked paprika then mix the ingredients well.
- ➢ In a pan, sauté a drizzle of olive oil.
- ➢ As soon as it is hot, sauté the artichokes for 10 minutes. Season with salt and pepper and put them on a plate.
- ➢ Take a non-stick pan, heat a little oil and cook for 2 minutes on each side and then add a little of artichokes and the cheddar cheese.
- ➢ Close the omelette, cook for another minute on each side and place it on a serving dish.
- ➢ Meanwhile, wash and chop parsley.
- ➢ Serve hot sprinkled with chopped parsley.

Baked feta and cherry tomatoes

Servings: 4 I Prep time: 10 minutes I Cook time. 15 minutes
Nutrition facts per serving: calories: 210; carbs: 5 gr; protein: 15 gr; fat: 6 gr.

Ingredients
- ✓ 120 gr of feta
- ✓ 1 small onion
- ✓ 12 cherry tomatoes
- ✓ ½ tsp of dried oregano
- ✓ Olive oil, salt and pepper

Directions

- First, wash the cherry tomatoes and then cut them into 4 wedges.
- Peel and wash the small onion and then cut it into thin slices.
- Cut fete cheese into little pieces.
- Brush a baking sheet with olive oil.
- Place the feta pieces in the centre of the baking sheet.
- Now put the onion and cherry tomatoes.
- Season everything with oil, salt and pepper and then sprinkle with oregano.
- Bake in the oven at 180°c for 15 minutes.
- As soon as it is ready, take out of the oven, put the baked feta and tomatoes on a serving dish and serve.

Bell peppers and cheddar nuggets

Servings: 4 I Prep time: 10 minutes I Cook time: 15/20 minutes
Nutrition facts per serving: calories: 170; carbs: 7.7 gr; protein: 11 gr; fat: 7 gr.

Ingredients
- 8 long and small bell peppers
- 100 gr of cheddar cheese
- 2 tsp of oregano
- 1 tbsp of olive oil

Directions
- First, preheat the oven to 180° c.
- Cut off the top of the bell peppers and remove the cap, seeds, and internal filaments.
- Cut cheddar cheese into pieces.
- Place a piece of cheddar cheese in each pepper.
- Sprinkle with a bit of oregano.
- Place the peppers in the baking pan.
- Cook for 15/20 minutes circ.
- Cook until the bell peppers are completely cooked, and cheddar melted.
- Serve the bell peppers still hot.

Broccoli and courgettes eggs

Servings: 4 I Prep time: 10 minutes I Cook time: 10/15 minutes
Nutrition facts per serving: calories: 180; carbs: 5 gr; protein: 16 gr; fat: 4 gr.

Ingredients:
- 4 eggs
- 2 little courgettes
- 300 gr of broccoli (flowers only)
- 1 tsp of olive oil
- Salt and pepper

Directions
- First bring a pot of water to a boil.
- Cook the eggs in boiling water for at least 10 minutes.
- Always make sure that the eggs are completely covered with water.
- When cooked, place them in cold water to stop cooking and roll them on a smooth surface, gently squeezing them to break the shell.
- Shell them and cut them into wedges.
- In the meantime, wash the courgettes and cut them into slices.
- Extract only the flowers of the broccoli.
- Cook the vegetables on a pre-heated grill on both sides and when they are ready, place them on a plate with the eggs in the centre.
- Season everything with salt and pepper.
- You can serve your veggies eggs.

Chilli avocado eggs

Servings: 4 I Prep time: 10 minutes I Cook time: 15/20 minutes
Nutrition facts per serving: calories: 220; carbs: 5 gr; protein: 13 gr; fat: 14 gr.

Ingredients
- 4 large eggs
- 2 avocados
- 1 tbsp of chilli powder
- 10 gr of chopped chives
- Olive oil and salt

Directions
- First, preheat the oven to 180°c.
- Meanwhile, halve the avocado and remove the pulp and the central stone.
- Break the eggs and pour each of them in the middle of the avocado.
- Be very careful in this step, you have to make sure that the egg does not come out of the avocado.
- Bake in the oven for at least 15 minutes.
- Check for yourself which egg you like best.
- When eggs will be ready you can season with salt, chilli and finally chives.
- You can serve your chilli avocado eggs.

Coconut and cocoa pudding

Servings: 4 I Prep time: 10 minutes I Cook time: 1 minute
Nutrition facts per serving: calories: 150; carbs: 6.8 gr; protein: 10 gr; fat: 9 gr.

Ingredients
- ✓ 100 gr of coconut flour
- ✓ 70 ml of water
- ✓ 2 tbsp of coconut milk
- ✓ 2 tbsp of greek yogurt
- ✓ 10 gr of unsweetened cocoa powder

Directions
- ➤ Start by combining greek yogurt with coconut flour, water, coconut milk in a microwave-safe bowl.
- ➤ Stir well and add the cocoa powder too.
- ➤ Microwave for 45 seconds.
- ➤ Add additional coconut milk, or water, if necessary.
- ➤ You can serve pudding.

Coconut pistachios and blackberries bowl

Servings: 4 I Prep time: 10 minutes I Cook time: -
Nutrition facts per serving: calories: 180; carbs: 8 gr; protein: 10 gr; fat: 11 gr.

Ingredients
- ✓ 400 gr of greek yogurt
- ✓ 1 teaspoon of stevia
- ✓ 300 gr of blackberries
- ✓ 40 gr of chopped pistachios
- ✓ 2 tbsp of coconut grains

Directions
- ➤ First, wash and dry the blackberries and put 200 gr of them in the blender glass together with the stevia, and yogurt.
- ➤ Blend at maximum speed until you get a creamy and lump-free mixture.
- ➤ As soon as it is ready, put the mixture in 4 bowls.
- ➤ Put the remaining blackberries, chopped pistachios, coconut grains on top of the mixture and serve.

Grapefruit and berries yogurt salad

Servings: 4 I Prep time: 10 minutes + 30 minutes of rest in the fridge I Cook time: 10 minutes
Nutrition facts per serving: calories: 120; carbs: 8 gr; protein: 5 gr; fat: 6 gr.

Ingredients
- ✓ 1 pink grapefruit
- ✓ 100 gr of mixed berries
- ✓ 1 tsp of liquid stevia
- ✓ 200 gr of greek yogurt
- ✓ 2 tsp of ground cinnamon

Directions

- ➤ First, peel the grapefruit.
- ➤ Divide it into wedges and place them in a bowl.
- ➤ Squeeze a bit of lime juice into a small bowl. Add the stevia and mix well.
- ➤ Wash and dry berries and place them in the same bowl of grapefruit.
- ➤ Sprinkle the fruits with the lime sauce and mix everything gently.
- ➤ Transfer the fruit to the fridge to marinate for 30 minutes.
- ➤ After 30 minutes, take the fruit from the fridge and divide it into 4 bowls.
- ➤ Put the yogurt in a bowl and add the cinnamon.
- ➤ Mix well and then divide the yogurt into the 4 cups.
- ➤ You can serve your snacks.

Paprika parmesan fries

Servings: 4 I Prep time: 10 minutes I Cook time: 10 minutes
Nutrition facts per serving: calories: 180; carbs: 2 gr; protein: 14 gr; fat 8 gr.

Ingredients
- ✓ 200 gr of grated parmesan cheese
- ✓ 1 tsp of smoked paprika
- ✓ 1 tbsp of chopped parsley

Directions
- ➤ Start by preheating the oven to 190°c.
- ➤ Line a baking tray with parchment paper and form piles with the cheese, making sure to leave enough space between one pile and another.
- ➤ If one tray is not enough, divide the cheese into two trays.
- ➤ Sprinkle the parmesan with parmesan and smoked paprika.
- ➤ Place the pan in the oven and cook for 8-10 minutes, making sure that the cheese does not burn.
- ➤ Let cool and then serve your parmesan fries.

Pineapple and strawberry salad

Servings: 4 I Prep time: 10 minutes + 30 minutes in the fridge fro marinating I Cook time: 10 minutes
Nutrition facts per serving: calories: 100; carbs: 6 gr; protein: 5 gr; fat: 6 gr.

Ingredients
- ✓ Half a pineapple
- ✓ 20 strawberries

- ✓ 1 tsp of stevia
- ✓ 200 ml of unsweetened orange juice
- ✓ 4 tbsp of greek yogurt

Directions

➢ Peel the pineapple, wash the pulp, and then cut into cubes.
➢ Wash the strawberries and then cut them into slices.
➢ Put the fruit in a bowl, sprinkle it with the stevia and then the orange juice.
➢ Mix gently and then transfer the bowl to the fridge to marinate for 30 minutes.
➢ As soon as it is ready, place it in 4 individual cups and serve with a tablespoon of greek yogurt for each.

Pistachio and soy avocado chips

Servings: 4 I Prep time: 10 minutes I Cook time: 15/20 minutes
Nutrition facts per serving: calories: 180; carbs: 5 gr; protein: 10 gr; fat: 8 gr.

Ingredients

- ✓ 1 avocado
- ✓ 50 gr of soy flour
- ✓ 70 ml water
- ✓ 40 gr of chopped pistachios
- ✓ Salt and pepper to taste

Directions

➢ First, halve the avocado.
➢ Wash it and remove the central stone.
➢ Cut the avocado into slices that are not too thin. In a bowl, dissolve the soy flour with the water, mixing well.
➢ Season with salt and pepper and a pinch of nutmeg. Pour the chopped pistachios in another dish.
➢ Pass the avocado slices first in the soy flour batter, then in the pistachios and arrange them on a baking sheet lined with parchment paper.
➢ Once all the avocado slices have been breaded, bake them in a static oven at 160° c for 15/20 minutes, seasoning them first with a drop of oil to make them golden.
➢ Once ready, serve still hot the avocado chips.

Orange and nuts salad

Servings: 4 I Prep time: 10 minutes I Cook time: -
Nutrition facts per serving: calories: 130; carbs: 7 gr; protein: 3 gr; fat: 12 gr.

Ingredients

- ✓ 2 oranges
- ✓ 20 gr of sliced almonds
- ✓ 20 gr of chopped pistachios
- ✓ 20 gr of chopped pecans
- ✓ 2 tbsp of apple cider vinegar
- ✓ Olive oil, salt and pepper

Directions

➢ First, peel the oranges, wash them, grate the zest, and then cut them into slices.
➢ Arrange the orange slices in a circle on a serving dish.
➢ Put oil, salt, pepper, apple cider vinegar, and the orange zest in a bowl and mix with a fork.
➢ Sprinkle the oranges with this emulsion.
➢ Now put the almonds, pistachios, and pecans on top of the oranges and serve your snack salad.

Red berries and nuts granola

Servings: 4 I Prep time: 10 minutes I Cook time: 60 minutes
Nutrition facts per serving: calories: 200; carbs: 5.8 gr; protein: 12 gr; fat: 15.

Ingredients

- ✓ 60 gr of chopped hazelnuts
- ✓ 60 gr of chopped walnuts
- ✓ 40 gr of almond flakes
- ✓ 160 gr of red berries
- ✓ 20 gr of low-carb maple syrup

Directions

➢ First, put the almond flakes, chopped hazelnuts and walnuts in a bowl.
➢ Wash and dry the red berries and put them in the bowl.
➢ Add the low-carb maple syrup, a tablespoon of olive oil and 4 tablespoons of cold water and mix everything well.
➢ Now take a baking sheet and cover it with parchment paper.
➢ Spread the mixture into the pan and cook in the oven at 160 °C for 60 minutes.
➢ Every 20 minutes remember to mix the granola to prevent burning.
➢ Just cooked, take it out of the oven and let it cool.
➢ Break the granola with your hands and serve.

Strawberry and almond salad

Servings: 4 I Prep time: 10 minutes I Cook time: -
Nutrition facts per serving: calories: 110; carbs: 6 gr; protein: 4 gr; fat: 7 gr.

Ingredients

- ✓ 400 gr of strawberries
- ✓ 1 lime
- ✓ 1 teaspoon of stevia
- ✓ 1 teaspoon of vanilla powder
- ✓ 2 tbsp of chopped almonds

Directions

- ➤ First, wash and dry the strawberries. Cut it into pieces.
- ➤ Put the strawberries in a bowl.
- ➤ Squeeze the lime and strain the juice into the bowl with the strawberries.
- ➤ Add the stevia and vanilla and mix everything gently.
- ➤ Put the strawberries in the fridge to macerate for an hour.
- ➤ Now take the strawberries, put them in serving bowls, decorated with chopped almonds and serve.

Walnuts and artichokes triangles

Servings: 4 I Prep time: 10 minutes I Cook time: 15 minutes
Nutrition facts per serving: calories: 280; carbs: 8 gr; protein: 18 gr; fat: 10 gr.

Ingredients
- ✓ 1 roll of low-carb shortcrust pastry
- ✓ 4 artichokes
- ✓ 10 walnuts
- ✓ 2 tbsp of soy sauce
- ✓ 100 ml cooking cream

Directions

- ➤ First, peel the walnuts and chop very coarsely.
- ➤ Clean and peel the artichokes, sauté them slowly in a pan with a little oil, 2 tablespoons of soy sauce, a bit of finely chopped parsley, 2 chopped bay leaf and chopped walnuts, for half an hour.
- ➤ When the mixture is well browned, turn off and pass in the mixer leaving it quite coarse and add the cooking cream to emulsify.
- ➤ It is necessary to obtain a medium consistency, neither liquid nor dry, suitable for filling the dough.
- ➤ After having cut out some triangles of dough fill them with the mixture, close them well and sprinkle them with the fat brush with a cream obtained by working a bit of butter with a fork.
- ➤ Bake on a baking pan for 15 minutes at 180 °c.
- ➤ Serve still hot.

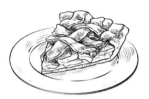

Desserts and baked good recipes

Almond and cocoa cake

Servings: 4 I Prep time: 10 minutes I Cook time: 30 minutes
Nutrition facts per serving: calories: 200; carbs: 6 gr; protein: 14 gr; fat: 10 gr.

Ingredients
- ✓ 300 gr of almond flour
- ✓ 150 unsweetened almond milk
- ✓ 50 gr of unsweetened cocoa powder
- ✓ 150 ml of melted butter

Directions
- ➢ First, preheat the oven to 180° c.
- ➢ Meanwhile, prepare the cake dough.
- ➢ Separate the yolks and egg whites, beat the egg whites until stiff in a bowl, and set aside.
- ➢ Beat the egg yolks in another bowl.
- ➢ Add the butter and a bit of almond milk.
- ➢ Gradually add the almond flour and cocoa powder, mixing and blending the mixture well.
- ➢ Pour in the milk, previously kept aside.
- ➢ At the end, carefully add the whipped egg whites.
- ➢ Mix and incorporate them gently.
- ➢ Pour the mixture into a cake mould previously greased with a bit of oil.
- ➢ Cook in a convection oven for about 30 minutes.
- ➢ Always check the cooking with a toothpick.
- ➢ Serve the cake as soon as it has cooled slightly.

Almond coconut and pistachio muffins

Servings: 4 I Prep time: 10 minutes I Cook time: 30 minutes
Nutrition facts per serving: calories: 290; carbs: 13 gr; protein: 14 gr; fat: 18 gr; fibre: 5 gr.

Ingredients
- ✓ 120 gr of coconut flour
- ✓ 120 gr of almond flour
- ✓ 4 tbsp of finely chopped pistachios
- ✓ 200 ml of unsweetened coconut milk
- ✓ 1 lemon zest
- ✓ Olive oil and salt

Directions
- ➢ First, peel and chop very finely 4 tbsp of pistachios.
- ➢ Meanwhile wash and take a lemon zest.
- ➢ In a large bowl pour all the dry ingredients (almond and coconut flours, lemon zest, chopped pistachios, 1 tsp of baking powder and a pinch of salt) and mix everything well.
- ➢ Then add the coconut milk the oil and mix again until you get a soft and homogeneous consistency.
- ➢ Transfer the mixture into muffin moulds.
- ➢ Bake your muffins at 170°c for about 30 minutes.
- ➢ When they will be ready, let muffins cool and serve.

Almond yogurt and berries

Servings: 4 I Prep time: 10 minutes I Cook time: 15 minutes
Nutrition facts per serving: calories: 230; carbs:9 gr protein: 14 gr fat: 8 gr.

Ingredients
- ✓ 80 gr of almond flour
- ✓ 300 ml of greek yogurt
- ✓ 1 tbsp of stevia powder
- ✓ 4 tbsp of chopped hazelnuts
- ✓ 400 gr of mixed berries

Directions
- ➢ Start by preheating the oven to 160° c.
- ➢ In a fairly large bowl, combine the almond flour, the stevia, a tbsp of olive oil, hazelnuts and a pinch of salt.
- ➢ Mix the ingredients with your hands until many grains have formed.
- ➢ Pour the mixture into a baking tray covered with parchment paper and cook for 12 minutes, stirring the mixture from time to time to prevent it from burning.
- ➢ In the meantime, move on to preparing the cake bases.
- ➢ Wash and dry the berries and then chop them into small cubes.
- ➢ Put half of soy yogurt and strawberries in 4 glasses and then put them in the fridge to rest.
- ➢ When the chopped almonds are cooked, remove it from the oven and let it cool.
- ➢ As soon as it is cold, take the glasses with the berries and yogurt from the fridge and sprinkle them with the granola and then serve.

Avocado and orange ice cream

Servings: 4 I Prep time: 10 minutes + 1 hour in the freezer I Cook time: -
Nutrition facts per serving: calories: 180; carbs: 6 gr, protein: 4 gr, fat: 13 gr.

Ingredients
✓ 400 gr of avocado pulp
✓ 1 orange
✓ 200 ml of unsweetened almond milk
✓ 2 tbsp of powdered stevia

Directions
➢ First, peel and cut the avocado in two. Remove the stone, then wash and dry it.
➢ Take 400 gr of pulp and cut into pieces.
➢ Put the avocado in the blender glass.
➢ Add the almond milk and blend the ingredients at medium speed until you get a smooth and homogeneous mixture.
➢ Add the stevia and the juice of the filtered strips orange.
➢ Continue to blend for another minute so that all the ingredients are well blended.
➢ Put the mixture in a container and put it in the freezer for an hour.
➢ Then transfer the mixture to the ice cream maker following the times indicated in the ice cream maker to prepare the ice cream.
➢ As soon as it's ready, put the ice cream back in the freezer to harden it and then serve it.

Blackberry vanilla and soy ice cream

Servings: 4 I Prep time: 10 minutes + 4 hours in the freezer I Cook time: -
Nutrition facts per serving: calories: 100; carbs: 6.5 gr; protein: 6 gr; fat: 5 gr; fibre: 3 gr.

Ingredients
✓ 80 ml of unsweetened soy milk
✓ 400 gr of blackberries
✓ 2 tbsp of powdered stevia
✓ 1 tsp of vanilla powder

Directions
➢ Firstly, quickly rinse the blackberries in cold water, drain and lay them out to dry on a paper towel.
➢ Blend the sot milk with the blackberries, vanilla powder, and stevia in a blender until the mixture is homogeneous and filter it through a fine-mesh strainer.
➢ Mix and pour the mixture into the ice cream moulds.

➢ Place the stick in the centre and freeze in the freezer for at least 4 hours.
➢ Turn out the ice cream and serve.

Blueberry and ginger ice cream

Servings: 4 I Prep time: 10 minutes + 4 hours in the freezer I Cook time: -
Nutrition facts per serving: calories: 70; carbs: 5 gr; protein: 2 gr; fat: 1 gr.

Ingredients
✓ 400 ml of semi-skimmed milk
✓ 300 gr of blueberries
✓ 2 tsp of powdered stevia
✓ 2 tbsp of minced ginger

Directions
➢ Start by rinsing the blueberries in cold water. After that, drain and lay them out to dry on a paper towel.
➢ Peel wash and mince ginger.
➢ Blend the milk with the blueberries, ginger, and stevia in a blender until the mixture is homogeneous, and filter it through a fine-mesh strainer
➢ Mix and pour the mixture into the ice cream moulds.
➢ Freeze for at least 4 hours after inserting the stick in the centre.
➢ Remove the ice cream from the freezer and serve.

Cinnamon and pumpkin cake

Servings: 4 I Prep time: 10 minutes I Cook time: 60 minutes
Nutrition facts per serving: calories: 260, carbs: 7.8 gr; protein: 11 gr; fat: 22 gr.

Ingredients
✓ 120 gr of already cleaned pumpkin pulp
✓ 200 gr of almond flour
✓ 4 tbsp of olive oil
✓ 60 ml of almond milk
✓ 1 tsp of powdered cinnamon
✓ Backing powder + pinch of salt

Directions
➢ First, use a spoon to remove all of the seeds and internal filaments from the pumpkin.
➢ Remove the peel from the pumpkin and cut it into 3 cm about thick slices with a sharp knife.
➢ 1 cup cleaned pumpkin, weighed, and sliced on a baking sheet lined with parchment paper

- ➢ Bake for 20 minutes at 180° C in a static oven, then remove and cool.
- ➢ You can now proceed to making the cake dough. In the food processor, blend the roasted pumpkin until smooth.
- ➢ Pour the almond flour, cinnamon, a tsp of baking powder and a pinch of salt into a bowl.
- ➢ Stir in the pumpkin puree, olive oil, and almond milk with a wooden spoon until well combined.
- ➢ Pour the batter into a 22-cm-diameter parchment-lined cake pan.
- ➢ Bake your pumpkin cake in a static oven at 170°c for about 40 minutes.
- ➢ Check the cooking and when cake will be done, remove from the oven and let cool completely before serving.

Coconut and strawberries ice cream

Servings: 4 I Prep time: 10 minutes + 4 hours in the freezer I Cook time: -
Nutrition facts per serving: calories: 120; carbs: 5 gr; protein: 8 gr; fat: 4 gr.

Ingredients
- ✓ 40 ml of unsweetened coconut milk
- ✓ 300 gr of strawberries
- ✓ 20 ml of sugar free whipped cream
- ✓ 2 tbsp of stevia

Directions
- ➢ Firstly, quickly rinse the strawberries in cold water, drain and lay them out to dry on a paper towel.
- ➢ Blend the coconut milk with the strawberries and the stevia in a blender until the mixture is homogeneous and filter it through a fine-mesh strainer to eliminate the seeds.
- ➢ Add the soy milk whipped cream, mix and pour the mixture into the ice cream moulds.
- ➢ Place the stick in the centre and freeze in the freezer for at least 4 hours.
- ➢ Turn out the ice cream and serve.

Coconut lime and avocado cream

Servings: 4 I Prep time: 10 minutes + 1 hour in the freezer I Cook time: -
Nutrition facts per serving: calories: 190; carbs: 6.5 gr, protein: 4 gr, fat: 14 gr.

Ingredients
- ✓ 400 gr of avocado pulp
- ✓ 1 lime
- ✓ 200 ml of unsweetened coconut milk

- ✓ 2 tbsp of powdered stevia
- ✓ 1 tbsp of coconut flour

Directions
- ➢ First, peel and cut the avocado in two. Remove the central core, then wash and dry it.
- ➢ Take 400 gr of pulp and cut into pieces.
- ➢ Put the avocado in the blender glass.
- ➢ Add the coconut flour and milk and blend the ingredients at medium speed until you get a smooth and homogeneous mixture.
- ➢ Add the stevia and the juice of the filtered lime.
- ➢ Continue to blend for another minute so that all the ingredients are well blended.
- ➢ Put the mixture in a container and put it in the freezer for an hour.
- ➢ Then transfer the mixture to the ice cream maker following the times indicated in the ice cream maker to prepare the ice cream.
- ➢ As soon as it's ready, put the ice cream back in the freezer to harden it and then serve it.

Cottage cheese and peanuts mousse

Servings: 4 I Prep time: 10 minutes I Cook time: 10-15 minutes
Nutrition facts per serving: calories: 210; carbs: 4 gr; protein: 18 gr; fat: 6 gr.

Ingredients
- ✓ 200 gr of ricotta cheese
- ✓ 1 orange
- ✓ 1 tsp of vanilla extract
- ✓ 1 tsp of stevia
- ✓ 2 tbsp of chopped peanuts

Directions
- ➢ First, wash and dry the orange, grate the zest, and strain the juice into a saucepan.
- ➢ Put a glass of water in the saucepan and cook them with the stevia until you have obtained a sort of syrup.
- ➢ Put the cottage cheese in a bowl and add the vanilla extract.
- ➢ Stir and mix well and then add the orange syrup
- ➢ With the help of a manual whisk, mix the ingredients until you have obtained a fairly smooth and compact mixture.
- ➢ Put the mousse in the glasses, decorate it with the grated orange zest and keep the mousse in the fridge until you need to serve it.
- ➢ When you will serve the mousse, pour over a bit of chopped peanuts, and serve.

Pineapple and almond cake

Servings: 4 I Prep time: 10 minutes I Cook time: 35 minutes
Nutrition facts per serving: calories: 190; carbs: 6.8 gr; protein: 7 gr; fat: 10 gr.

Ingredients
- ✓ 120 gr of fresh pineapple pulp
- ✓ 100 gr of almond flour
- ✓ 3 tbsp of powdered stevia
- ✓ 30 ml of melted butter
- ✓ 100 ml of almond milk
- ✓ Backing soda + salt

Directions
- ➢ You can start preparing the cake dough.
- ➢ Mix the almond flour, stevia 1 tsp of baking soda, a pich of salt, and 1 tsp vanilla extract in a bowl, and then add the melted butter and almond milk.
- ➢ Remove the pineapple pulp and the cut it into cubes and add them to the cake dough, mixing well to mix all the ingredients.
- ➢ Add other almond milk if it is necessary.
- ➢ Line a pan with parchment paper and pour in the cake mixture.
- ➢ Level the surface well and decorate it with the pineapple slices, then brush them with a bit of oil.
- ➢ Bake in a static oven at 180°c for 35 minutes, doing the toothpick test before taking it out of the oven to check that it is cooked.
- ➢ If it is not cooked, let it cook for another five minutes.
- ➢ When cake will be removed from the oven, let cool completely and serve.

Pistachio cookies

Servings: 4 I Prep time: 10 minutes I Cook time: 10-15 minutes
Nutrition facts per serving: calories: 120; carbs: 4.5 gr; protein: 10 gr; fat: 10 gr.

Ingredients
- ✓ 6 tbsp of almond flour
- ✓ 2 tbsp of chopped pistachios
- ✓ 2 egg whites
- ✓ 1 tbsp of softened butter

Directions
- ➢ You can start this recipe with preheating the oven to 180°c.
- ➢ Meanwhile, in a bowl, beat the egg whites until stiff.

- ➢ After they are whipped, you can add all the other ingredients and mix, until you get a homogeneous mixture.
- ➢ Add the softened butter and mix again.
- ➢ If the dough is too dry, you can always add more egg white a little at a time.
- ➢ If it turns out to be too liquid, you can add a little almond flour.
- ➢ Line a baking sheet with parchment paper.
- ➢ Start now to create the cookies of the shape you prefer.
- ➢ After placing the cookies in the pan, bake them for 10/12 minutes.
- ➢ Bake the cookies until golden brown.
- ➢ Serve when they have cooled slightly.

Raspberries ice cream

Servings: 4 I Prep time: 10 minutes + 4 hours in the fridge I Cook time:-
Nutrition facts per serving: calories: 90; carbs: 3 gr; protein:8 gr; fat: 4 gr.

Ingredients
- ✓ 400 gr of raspberries
- ✓ 60 ml of sugar free almond milk
- ✓ 40 ml of sugar free whipped cream
- ✓ 2 tbsp of stevia

Directions
- ➢ Firstly, quickly rinse the raspberries in cold water, drain and lay them out to dry on a paper towel.
- ➢ Blend the almond milk with the raspberries and the stevia in a blender until the mixture is homogeneous and filter it through a fine-mesh strainer to eliminate the seeds.
- ➢ Add the soy milk whipped cream, mix, and pour the mixture into the ice cream moulds.
- ➢ Place the stick in the centre and freeze in the freezer for at least 4 hours.
- ➢ Turn out the ice cream and serve.

Raspberries in dark chocolate sauce

Servings: 4 I Prep time: 10 minutes I Cook time: 10-15 minutes
Nutrition facts per serving: calories: 170; carbs: 8 gr; protein: 4 gr; fat: 5 gr.

Ingredients
- ✓ 400 ml of low-carb whipped cream
- ✓ The zest of a grated orange
- ✓ 100 gr of 90% dark chocolate
- ✓ 300 gr of raspberries
- ✓ 1 tbsp of chopped mint leaves

Directions
➢ Start by finely chopping the dark chocolate.
➢ Pour the whipped cream into a saucepan.
➢ Put the saucepan on the stove and bring the cream to the limit of the boil.
➢ Then remove the pot from the heat, add the chocolate and let it melt slowly.
➢ Wash raspberries, let them dry and arrange them in a deep dish in a single layer, and perfume them with the orange zest.
➢ Then mix the cream again with a spatula until all the chocolate is well melted and the sauce is smooth and silky.
➢ Pour the sauce over the raspberries, decorate with a few mint leaves, and serve.

Redberry and lemon popsicles

Servings: 4 I Prep time: 10 minutes + 4 hours in the freezer I Cook time:-
Nutrition facts per serving: calories: 35; carbs: 2 gr; protein: 1 gr; fat: 2 gr.

Ingredients
✓ 80 ml of sugar free almond milk
✓ 1 lemon
✓ 20 red berries
✓ 2 tsp of stevia powder

Directions
➢ First, wash and let dry red berries
➢ Wash and dry the lemon, grate the zest, and filter the juice into the glass of a blender.
➢ Also add the almond milk, red berries, stevia, and zest.
➢ Blend everything at maximum speed until you get a smooth and homogeneous mixture.
➢ Take the popsicle moulds and transfer the mixture inside.
➢ Put in the freezer and let it rest for 4 hours.
➢ After 4 hours you can take the popsicles and serve them.

Oat vanilla and wild strawberries ice cream

Servings: 4 I Prep time: 10 minutes + 4 hours in the freezer I Cook time: -
Nutrition facts per serving: calories: 124; carbs: 5 gr; protein: 10 gr; fat: 6 gr.

Ingredients
✓ 60 ml of unsweetened oat milk
✓ 4 tbsp of soy milk whipped cream
✓ 2 tbsp of powdered stevia

✓ 400 gr of wild strawberries
✓ 1 tsp of vanilla extract

Directions
➢ First, quickly wash the wild strawberries in cold water, drain and lay them out to dry on a paper towel.
➢ Blend the oat milk with the wild strawberries and the stevia in a blender until the mixture is homogeneous and filter it through a fine-mesh strainer to eliminate the seeds.
➢ Add the soy milk whipped cream, vanilla extract and mix and pour the mixture into the ice cream moulds.
➢ Place the stick in the centre and freeze in the freezer for at least 4 hours.
➢ Turn out the ice cream and serve.

Soy and coconut cake

Servings: 4 I Prep time: 10 minutes I Cook time: 30 minutes
Nutrition facts per serving: calories: 160; carbs: 4 gr; protein: 14 gr; fat: 10 gr.

Ingredients
✓ 200 gr of soy flour
✓ 100 gr of coconut flour
✓ 150 ml of melted coconut oil
✓ 2 eggs
✓ 2 tbsp of stevia powder

Directions
➢ First, preheat the oven to 180°c.
➢ Meanwhile, prepare the cake dough.
➢ Separate the yolks and egg whites, beat the egg whites until stiff in a bowl, and set aside.
➢ Beat the egg yolks in another bowl with the stevia.
➢ Add the melted coconut oil.
➢ Gradually add the two flours, mixing and blending the mixture well.
➢ Pour in the milk, previously kept aside.
➢ At the end, carefully add the whipped egg whites.
➢ Mix and incorporate them gently.
➢ Pour the mixture into a cake mould previously greased with a bit of olive oil.
➢ Cook in a convection oven for about 30 minutes.
➢ Always check the cooking with a toothpick.
➢ Serve the cake as soon as it has cooled slightly.

Strawberry and cheese pie

Servings: 4 I Prep time: 10 minutes + 5 minutes in the freezer I Cook time: -

Nutrition facts per serving: calories: 90; carbs: 5 gr; protein: 8 gr; fat: 4gr.

Ingredients
- ✓ 120 gr of melted coconut oil
- ✓ 2 tsp of orange juice
- ✓ 120 gr of sugar free cream cheese
- ✓ 4 tbsp of powdered stevia
- ✓ 300 gr of strawberries

Directions
- ➤ First, melt the coconut oil in a low-power microwave safe bowl.
- ➤ Check it every 10-20 seconds because you will need to get a slightly warm melted coconut oil.
- ➤ Stir it often until it is completely dissolved.
- ➤ Meanwhile, wash and let dry strawberries.
- ➤ In a medium bowl, melted coconut oil then add the cream cheese and mix well.
- ➤ Also add the stevia, strawberries, and orange juice.
- ➤ Mix all the ingredients well.
- ➤ Pour the mixture into small silicone moulds and put them in the freezer for at least 4 hours, until the cakes have hardened.
- ➤ To serve these cakes, take them out of the freezer 5 minutes before serving.
- ➤ Remove them from the silicone moulds and place them in a small tray, plate, or small paper cups.
- ➤ Serve very cold.

Vanilla and pecans cheesy mousse

Servings: 4 I Prep time: 10 minutes + 1 hour in the fridge I Cook time: -
Nutrition facts per serving: calories: 240; carbs: 8.7 gr; protein: 16 gr; fat: 12 gr.

Ingredients
- ✓ 200 gr of low-carb cream cheese
- ✓ 200 ml of unsweetened coconut milk
- ✓ 1 teaspoon of vanilla extract
- ✓ 5 tbsp of chopped pecans
- ✓ 2 tbsp of stevia powder
- ✓ Pinch of salt

Directions
- ➤ First, take a bowl and put the cream cheese inside.
- ➤ With an electric mixer, start working the cheese until you have obtained a light and fluffy cream.
- ➤ Set the mixer to minimum speed and add the vanilla extract first and then the coconut milk.
- ➤ While continuing to mix, add the sweetener and stir until well blended.
- ➤ Now add the chopped pecans and a pinch of salt, increase the speed of the mixer to the maximum

and continue to mix for another 2 minutes, or in any case until you have obtained a soft and homogeneous mixture.
- ➤ Put the mousse to rest in the fridge for an hour and then serve it in four glasses.

Walnuts and ginger sauce strawberries

Servings: 4 I Prep time: 10 minutes I Cook time: -
Nutrition facts per serving: calories: 160; carbs: 9 gr; protein: 4 gr; fat: 9 gr.

Ingredients
- ✓ 200 ml of low-carb whipped cream
- ✓ 300 gr of strawberries
- ✓ 2 tbsp chopped walnuts
- ✓ 1 piece of fresh ginger
- ✓ 2 tbsp of grated orange zest

Directions
- ➤ First, peel and finely chop walnuts.
- ➤ Peel, wash and chop a piece of ginger piece too.
- ➤ Pour the whipped cream into a saucepan.
- ➤ Put the saucepan on the stove and bring the cream to the limit of the boil.
- ➤ Then remove the pot from the heat, add the ginger and walnuts and swirl the pot to submerge it completely and let it melt slowly.
- ➤ Meanwhile, wash the strawberries removing the stalk.
- ➤ Cut them into little pieces and arrange them in a deep dish in a single layer and add the orange zest.
- ➤ Then mix the cream again until is smooth and silky.
- ➤ Pour the sauce over the strawberries and serve.

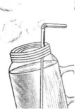

Smoothie recipes

Almond and berries smoothie

Servings: 4 I Prep time: 10 minutes I Cook time: -
Nutrition facts per serving: calories: 100; carbs:
6 gr; protein: 5 gr; fat: 3 gr.

Ingredients
- ✓ 300 ml of unsweetened almond milk
- ✓ 300 gr of mixed berries
- ✓ 2 tbsp of chopped almonds

Directions
- ➤ First, wash and dry the berries.
- ➤ Put the berries, chopped almonds and almond milk in the bowl of the mixer.
- ➤ Blend all the ingredients together with the blender on high speed.
- ➤ When the mixture is homogeneous and well blended, turn off the mixer, mix everything with a spatula or a wooden spoon and pour the smoothie into 4 glasses.
- ➤ Serve your smoothie.

Almond and pineapple smoothie

Servings: 4 I Prep time: 10 minutes I Cook time: -
Nutrition facts per serving: calories: 120; carbs:
8 gr; protein: 5 gr; fat: 6 gr.

Ingredients
- ✓ 200 gr of pineapple pulp
- ✓ 400 ml of unsweetened almond milk
- ✓ 1 teaspoon of cinnamon
- ✓ 1 teaspoon of stevia
- ✓ 1 tsp of chopped almonds

Directions
- ➤ First, wash and dry the pineapple pulp and then cut it into pieces.
- ➤ Put the pineapple pieces in the blender glass along with the cinnamon and stevia.
- ➤ Blend everything for a few seconds and then add the almond milk.
- ➤ Blend again for a few seconds and then add the ice cubes.
- ➤ Continue to blend until you get a thick and creamy mixture.
- ➤ Pour the smoothie into glasses, pour over with chopped almonds and serve.

Avocado and lime smoothie

Servings: 4 I Prep time: 10 minutes I Cook time: -
Nutrition facts per serving: calories: 180; carbs:
6 gr; protein: 7 gr; fat: 12 gr.

Ingredients:
- ✓ 1 avocado
- ✓ 300 ml of unsweetened almond milk
- ✓ Half a lime
- ✓ A tsp of stevia
- ✓ A tsp of vanilla powder

Directions
- ➤ First, peel and wash the avocado. Remove the stone and then cut the pulp into pieces.
- ➤ Put the avocado pulp into a blender glass. Add the almond milk, vanilla, and stevia.
- ➤ Turn on the blender and blend everything at maximum speed for one minute.
- ➤ Now add the ice cubes and lime juice and blend again until you get a thick and homogeneous mixture.
- ➤ Transfer the shake into the glasses, add the straws,
- ➤ You can serve your smoothie.

Berries and coconut smoothie

Servings: 4 I Prep time: 10 minutes I Cook time: -
Nutrition facts per serving: calories: 60; carbs: 5 gr;
protein: 2 gr; fat: 3 gr.

Ingredients
- ✓ 60 gr of blueberries
- ✓ 60 gr of cranberries
- ✓ 60 gr of raspberries
- ✓ 300 ml of unsweetened coconut milk
- ✓ 1 tsp of stevia

Directions
- ➤ First, wash the blueberries, cranberries, and raspberries and then let them drain.
- ➤ Now put the berries in the blender glass.
- ➤ Add the coconut milk, ice, and stevia.
- ➤ Turn on the blender and blend until you get a creamy mixture.
- ➤ Pour the smoothie into 4 glasses and serve.

Blackberry avocado and ginger smoothie

Servings: 4 I Prep time: 10 minutes I Cook time: -
Nutrition facts per serving: calories: 210; carbs: 6
gr; protein: 8 gr; fat: 12 gr.

Ingredients:
- ✓ 1 avocado
- ✓ 400 ml of unsweetened almond milk
- ✓ 12 blackberries
- ✓ 1 lime
- ✓ 1 tsp of powdered ginger

Directions
- ➤ First, peel the avocado, remove the stone, and then cut the pulp into pieces.
- ➤ Wash and dry the blackberries and then cut them in half.
- ➤ Wash the lime and then grate the zest.
- ➤ Put the avocado pulp, blackberries, powdered ginger, stevia, almond milk, lime zest, and ice in the blender glass.
- ➤ Turn on the blender and blend until you get a thick and homogeneous mixture.
- ➤ Put the smoothie in the glasses, add a straw and serve.

Carrot and cucumber smoothie

Servings: 4 I Prep time: 10 minutes I Cook time: -
Nutrition facts per serving: calories: 120; carbs: 5 gr; protein: 7 gr; fat: 3 gr.

Ingredients
- ✓ 500 ml of unsweetened soy milk
- ✓ 1 cucumber
- ✓ 1 teaspoon of nutmeg

Directions
- ➤ Peel the cucumber. Wash it, dry it, and cut it into small pieces.
- ➤ Put the cucumber in the blender glass.
- ➤ Add the nutmeg, and soy milk.
- ➤ Blend everything at maximum speed until you get a thick and creamy mixture.
- ➤ Transfer the smoothie into the glasses, place the straws, and serve.

Chia seeds berries and avocado smoothie

Servings: 4 I Prep time: 10 minutes I Cook time: -
Nutrition facts per serving: calories: 220; carbs: 6 gr; protein: 6 gr; fat: 11 gr.

Ingredients
- ✓ 1 avocado
- ✓ 200 gr of berries
- ✓ ½ cup of unsweetened almond milk
- ✓ 2 tbsp of chia seeds

- ✓ 4 drops of liquid stevia

Directions
- ➤ First, wash and dry the berries.
- ➤ Peel, remove central stone and wash avocado, then cut the pulp into pieces.
- ➤ Put berries, avocado, oat milk, ice cubes, stevia and chia seeds inside the blender cup and operate it at maximum speed
- ➤ Blend everything until you get a creamy and homogeneous mixture.
- ➤ You can serve your smoothies.

Citrus and ginger smoothie

Servings: 4 I Prep time: 10 minutes I Cook time: -
Nutrition facts per serving: calories: 70; carbs: 7 gr; protein: 1 gr; fat: 0 gr.

Ingredients
- ✓ 1 lime
- ✓ 2 oranges
- ✓ 30 gr of grated ginger
- ✓ A teaspoon of vanilla extract
- ✓ 1 teaspoon of stevia

Directions
- ➤ First peel the lime and orange and divide the wedges.
- ➤ Put the fruit in the glass of the blender along with the stevia and vanilla.
- ➤ Run the blender and blend at high speed for one minute.
- ➤ Now add the ice cubes and ginger.
- ➤ Blend again until you get a thick and homogeneous mixture.
- ➤ Divide the smoothie into glasses, add the straws and serve.

Coconut and avocado smoothie

Servings: 4 I Prep time: 10 minutes I Cook time: -
Nutrition facts per serving: calories: 205; carbs: 7.5 gr; protein: 9 gr; fat: 14 gr.

Ingredients
- ✓ 1 avocado
- ✓ 300 ml of unsweetened coconut milk
- ✓ A pinch of cinnamon
- ✓ 1 tsp of stevia
- ✓ 1 tsp of coconut flour

Directions
- ➤ Start by peeling and washing the avocado. Then remove the stone and then cut the pulp into pieces.

➤ Put the avocado into a blender glass. Add the coconut milk, cinnamon, and stevia.
➤ Turn on the blender and blend everything at maximum speed for one minute.
➤ Now add the ice cubes and blend again until you get a thick and homogeneous mixture.
➤ Transfer the shake into the glasses, add the straws,
➤ Sprinkle with coconut flour and serve.

Coconut pistachio and strawberry smoothie

Servings: 4 I Prep time: 10 minutes I Cook time: -
Nutrition facts per serving: calories: 180; carbs: 8 gr; protein: 12 gr; fat: 8 gr.

Ingredients
✓ 300 ml of unsweetened coconut milk
✓ 400 gr of strawberries
✓ 1 teaspoon of stevia
✓ 1 teaspoon of powdered ginger
✓ 1 tbsp of chopped pistachios
Directions
➤ First, wash strawberries under running water.
➤ Then dry and halve them.
➤ Put the strawberries pieces in the blender glass.
➤ Add the coconut milk, ginger, ice cubes and stevia and blend everything at maximum speed.
➤ When you get a thick and homogeneous smoothie, turn off the blender and transfer the mixture into the glasses.
➤ Put the straws, decorated with chopped pistachios, and serve.

Coffee and cocoa smoothie

Servings: 4 I Prep time: 10 minutes I Cook time: -
Nutrition facts per serving: calories: 70; carbs: 5 gr; protein: 5 gr; fat: 2 gr.

Ingredients
✓ 300 ml of espresso coffee
✓ 1 tsp of stevia
✓ 2 glasses of unsweetened oat milk
✓ 4 tsp of bitter cocoa
✓ 1 tbsp of vanilla powder
Directions
➤ Put the espresso and the vanilla in the blender glass and leave to flavour for 10 minutes.
➤ After 10 minutes, add the stevia, oat milk, and ice.
➤ Turn on the blender and blend until you get a creamy and thick mixture.

➤ Put the smoothie in the glass.
➤ Sprinkle with bitter cocoa, add a straw and serve.

Cranberries and yogurt smoothie

Servings: 4 I Prep time: 10 minutes I Cook time: -
Nutrition facts per serving: calories: 130; carbs: 7 gr; protein: 9 gr; fat: 6 gr.

Ingredients
✓ 120 gr of cranberries
✓ 300 ml of coconut milk
✓ 200 gr of greek yogurt
✓ 1 teaspoon of stevia
✓ 1 teaspoon of vanilla essence
Directions
➤ Peel wash cranberries and then put it in the blender glass.
➤ Blend for 30 seconds at high speed.
➤ Add the yogurt and coconut milk and blend for another 30 seconds.
➤ Finally add the stevia, vanilla and ice and blend until everything is well blended.
➤ Put in the glasses, add the straws and some ice cubes, and serve.

Ginger and avocado smoothie

Servings: 4 I Prep time: 10 minutes I Cook time: -
Nutrition facts per serving: calories: 170; carbs: 7 gr; protein: 6 gr; fat: 8 gr.

Ingredients
✓ 1 little avocado
✓ 300 ml of soy milk
✓ 1 tbsp of fresh minced ginger
✓ 4 tbsp of orange juice
✓ 1 tsp of powdered cinnamon
Directions
➤ First, peel and wash the avocado and remove the central stone.
➤ Take the pulp and then cut it into small pieces.
➤ Wash and dry the ginger, then mince.
➤ Put the orange juice in the blender glass.
➤ Add the avocado pieces, cinnamon, soy milk and both fresh and powdered ginger.
➤ Blend everything at high speed, until you get a smooth and homogeneous mixture.
➤ Put the smoothie in 4 glasses, add a few ice cubes and serve.

Lime wild strawberry and mint smoothie

Servings: 4 I Prep time: 10 minutes I Cook time: -
Nutrition facts per serving: calories: 140; carbs: 6 gr; protein: 5 gr; fat: 7 gr.

Ingredients
- ✓ 20 wild strawberries
- ✓ 6 mint leaves
- ✓ 1 lime
- ✓ 1 tsp of stevia
- ✓ 1 glass of unsweetened almond milk

Directions
- ➢ First, wash and dry the wild strawberries and then cut them into pieces.
- ➢ Wash and dry the mint leaves.
- ➢ Wash the lime and then grate the zest.
- ➢ Put the wild strawberries pieces, mint, stevia, almond milk, lime zest, and ice in the blender glass.
- ➢ Turn on the blender and blend until you get a thick and homogeneous mixture.
- ➢ Put the smoothie in the glass, add a straw and serve.

Orange and blueberries smoothie

Servings: 4 I Prep time: 10 minutes I Cook time: -
Nutrition facts per serving: calories: 130; carbs: 5 gr; protein: 5 gr; fat: 7 gr.

Ingredients
- ✓ 1 big orange
- ✓ 20 blueberries
- ✓ A teaspoon of vanilla extract
- ✓ 1 teaspoon of stevia

Directions
- ➢ First wash blueberries and cut them in half
- ➢ Peel the orange and divide the wedges.
- ➢ Put the fruit in the glass of the blender along with the stevia and vanilla.
- ➢ Run the blender and blend at high speed for one minute.
- ➢ Now add the ice cubes and blend again until you get a thick and homogeneous mixture.
- ➢ Divide the smoothie into glasses, add the straws and serve.

Pineapple and ginger smoothie

Servings: 4 I Prep time: 10 minutes I Cook time: -
Nutrition facts per serving: calories: 190; carbs: 7 gr; protein: 7 gr; fat: 12 gr.

Ingredients

- ✓ 200 gr of pineapple pulp
- ✓ 1 avocado
- ✓ 400 ml of unsweetened soy milk
- ✓ 1 teaspoon of powdered ginger
- ✓ 1 teaspoon of stevia

Directions
- ➢ First, wash and dry the pineapple pulp and then cut it into pieces.
- ➢ Peel the avocado, wash it and remove the pulp and the central stone.
- ➢ Put the avocado and pineapple in the blender glass along with the powdered ginger and stevia.
- ➢ Blend everything for a few seconds and then add the soy milk.
- ➢ Blend again for a few seconds and then add the ice cubes.
- ➢ Continue to blend until you get a thick and creamy mixture.
- ➢ Pour the smoothie into glasses and serve.

Raspberry walnuts and yogurt smoothie

Servings: 4 I Prep time: 10 minutes I Cook time: -
Nutrition facts per serving: calories: 80; carbs: 4 gr; protein: 8 gr; fat: 3 gr.

Ingredients
- ✓ 300 gr of raspberries
- ✓ 100 ml of greek yogurt
- ✓ 1 tsp of vanilla extract
- ✓ Chopped walnuts to decorate

Directions
- ➢ First, wash and dry the raspberries and then cut halve.
- ➢ Put the berries in the blender glass.
- ➢ Add the yogurt, vanilla, and some ice cube.
- ➢ Turn on the blender and blend until you get a thick and creamy mixture.
- ➢ Put the smoothie into the glasses. Sprinkle with a little chopped walnuts and serve.

Soy avocado and cocoa smoothie

Servings: 4 I Prep time: 10 minutes I Cook time: -
Nutrition facts per serving: calories: 200; carbs: 7 gr; protein: 9 gr; fat: 12 gr.

Ingredients
- ✓ 2 avocados
- ✓ 1 tsp of stevia
- ✓ 100 gr of bitter cocoa
- ✓ 2 glasses of unsweetened soy milk

Directions

➢ Peel the avocados and remove the stone.
➢ Cut the pulp into small pieces and put it in the blender glass.
➢ Add the stevia, cocoa, soy milk, and some ice cubes.
➢ Turn on the blender and blend until you get a creamy and homogeneous mixture.
➢ Now put the smoothie in a glass, sprinkle with a little bitter cocoa, add the straw and serve.

Strawberry and oat smoothie

Servings: 4 I Prep time: 10 minutes I Cook time: -
Nutrition facts per serving: calories: 150; carbs: 8 gr; protein: 11 gr; fat: 6 gr.

Ingredients
✓ 300 ml of unsweetened oat milk
✓ 400 gr of strawberries
✓ 1 teaspoon of stevia
✓ 1 teaspoon of vanilla essence
✓ 1 tbsp of oat flakes

Directions
➢ Start by washing strawberries under running water.
➢ Then dry the strawberries and halve them.
➢ Put the strawberries pieces in the blender glass.
➢ Add the oat milk, vanilla essence, ice cubes and stevia and blend everything at maximum speed.
➢ When you get a thick and homogeneous smoothie, turn off the blender and transfer the mixture into the glasses.
➢ Put the straws, decorated with strawberry slices, pour over oat flakes, and serve.

Walnut cucumber and strawberry smoothie

Servings: 4 I Prep time: 10 minutes I Cook time: -
Nutrition facts per serving: calories: 190; carbs: 7 gr; protein: 12 gr; fat: 8 gr.

Ingredients
✓ 1 cucumber
✓ 400 ml of unsweetened almond milk
✓ 300 gr of strawberries
✓ 3 tbsp of chopped walnuts

Directions
➢ First, peel the cucumber.
➢ Wash and dry and then cut it into pieces.
➢ Wash and dry the strawberries too removing the stalk and then cut into little pieces.

➢ Put the cucumber pieces, strawberries pieces, chopped walnuts and almond milk in the bowl of the mixer.
➢ Blend all the ingredients together with the blender on high speed.
➢ When the mixture is homogeneous and well blended, turn off the mixer, mix everything with a spatula or a wooden spoon and pour the smoothie into 4 glasses.
➢ Serve your smoothies.

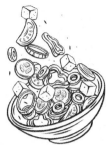

Only plant-based recipes

Almonds and courgettes bundles

Servings: 4 I Prep time: 10 minutes I Cook time: 30 minutes

Nutrition facts per serving: calories: 285; carbs 11 gr; protein 16 gr; fat 4 gr.

Ingredients
- ✓ 1 roll of homemade low-carb shortcrust pastry
- ✓ 1 big courgette
- ✓ 8 almonds
- ✓ 2 tbsp of low-carb soy sauce
- ✓ 100 ml of soymilk cream

Directions
- ➢ First, clean and peel the courgette cutting it into little slices.
- ➢ Rinse courgette slices under running water and let them dry.
- ➢ Sauté them slowly in a pan with a little oil, 2 tablespoons of soy sauce, and chopped almonds, for half an hour.
- ➢ When the mixture is well browned, turn off and pass in the mixer leaving it quite coarse and add the cream to emulsify.
- ➢ It is necessary to obtain a medium consistency, neither liquid nor dry, suitable for filling the dough.
- ➢ After having cut out some triangles of dough (from a round shape they come out comfortably 6) fill them with the mixture, close them well and sprinkle them with a little olive oil.
- ➢ Bake on a baking pan for half an hour at 180 ° c if you have a non-ventilated electric oven.
- ➢ Serve these bundles still hot.

Avocado lettuce and cauliflower salad

Servings: 4 I Prep time: 10 minutes I Cook time: 5 minutes

Nutrition facts per serving: calories: 230; carbs 9 gr; protein 8 gr; fat 12 gr.

Ingredients
- ✓ ½ cauliflower
- ✓ 100 gr of lettuce leaves
- ✓ 1 avocado
- ✓ 2 tablespoons of chia seeds

Directions
- ➢ First, clean and wash the cauliflower, divide it into florets and blanch them in lightly salted boiling water for about ten minutes, until the cauliflower begins to soften but is still firm enough.
- ➢ Wash and clean the lettuce leaves too and let them dry, then break them up.
- ➢ Drain it and if you like it, sauté it for 5 minutes in a pan with a drizzle of oil over a high flame to roast it slightly, then turn off the heat and let it cool.
- ➢ Meanwhile peel. Wash and remove the central stone from the avocado.
- ➢ Cut the pulp into slices.
- ➢ Combine the avocado slices, the cauliflower florets, the chopped lettuce, and the chia seeds in a bowl or serving dish.
- ➢ Season with the olive oil, a bit of apple cider vinegar and mix well before serving.

Bell peppers and tofu cream

Servings: 4 I Prep time: 10 minutes I Cook time: 25 minutes

Nutrition facts per serving: calories: 230; carbs 9 gr; protein 10 gr; fat 4 gr.

Ingredients
- ✓ 2 red peppers
- ✓ 2 white onions
- ✓ 200 gr of tomato pulp
- ✓ 80 gr of tofu
- ✓ Olive oil, salt and pepper

Directions
- ➢ First, halve the peppers, remove the cap, seeds, and white filaments, and then wash them.
- ➢ Cut them into slices.
- ➢ Peel the onions, wash, and chop them.
- ➢ Put a tablespoon of olive oil in a saucepan and then brown the onions for a couple of minutes.
- ➢ Add the tomato pulp and mix.
- ➢ Continue cooking for a couple of minutes and then add the sliced bell peppers.
- ➢ Add 350 ml of water and cook for 20 minutes.
- ➢ Meanwhile, rinse the tofu and pat it dry with absorbent paper.
- ➢ Cut it into cubes and sauté it for 3 minutes in a pan with a tablespoon of olive oil.
- ➢ Season with salt and pepper, turn off and set

aside.
- ➢ As soon as the peppers are cooked, turn off and blend everything with an immersion blender.
- ➢ Put the cream into four bowls.
- ➢ Add the tofu and when they have cooled, put the soups in the fridge until ready to serve.

Coconut milk and blueberries ice cream

Servings: 4 I Prep time: 10 minutes + 4 hours in the freezer I Cook time: -
Nutrition facts per serving: calories: 180; carbs 4.8 gr; protein 4 gr; fat 3 gr.

Ingredients
- ✓ 30 ml of coconut milk
- ✓ 300 gr of blueberries
- ✓ 20 ml of soy milk whipped cream
- ✓ 3 tbsp powdered stevia

Directions
- ➢ Firstly, quickly rinse the wild blueberries in cold water, drain and lay them out to dry on a paper towel.
- ➢ Blend the coconut milk with the blueberries and the brown sugar in a blender until the mixture is homogeneous and filter it through a fine-mesh strainer to eliminate the seeds.
- ➢ Add the soy milk whipped cream, mix, and pour the mixture into the ice cream moulds.
- ➢ Place the stick in the centre and freeze in the freezer for at least 4 hours.
- ➢ Turn out the ice cream and serve.

Herbs and soy cheese stuffed tomatoes

Servings: 4 I Prep time: 10 minutes I Cook time: 30 minutes
Nutrition facts per serving: calories: 190; carbs 7.8 gr; protein 7 gr; fat 3 gr.

Ingredients
- ✓ 10 piccadilly tomatoes
- ✓ 2 tbsp of mixed chopped fresh herbs
- ✓ 100 gr of soy cheese
- ✓ 2 tablespoons extra virgin olive oil

Directions
- ➢ Start with washing the tomatoes. Then, cut off the top and with a teaspoon, empty them of seeds.

- ➢ Let them drain upside down and in the meantime move on to preparing the filling.
- ➢ Wash all herbs then chop very coarsely.
- ➢ Fill the tomatoes with the herbs and soy cheese, using a teaspoon.
- ➢ Leave them to flavour in the fridge for at least 30 minutes.
- ➢ You can serve.

Lemon and almond tempeh

Servings: 4 I Prep time: 10 minutes + 30 minutes of marinating I Cook time: 5 minutes
Nutrition facts per serving: calories: 200; carbs 7 gr; protein 15 gr; fat 6 gr.

Ingredients
- ✓ 400 gr of tempeh
- ✓ 1 shallot
- ✓ 1 lemon
- ✓ 2 tbsp of almond flour
- ✓ Olive oil, salt and pepper

Directions
- ➢ First, rinse the tempeh and then pat it dry with a paper towel.
- ➢ Peel and wash the shallot and then cut it into slices.
- ➢ Wash and dry the lemon and then grate the zest.
- ➢ Put the tofu in a bowl together with the shallot, lemon zest, salt, pepper and two tablespoons of olive oil. Mix all ingredients to flavour.
- ➢ Leave to marinate for 30 minutes.
- ➢ After 30 minutes, drain the tempeh and cut it into cubes.
- ➢ Put 2 tbsp of almond flour on a plate and then pass the tempeh cubes.
- ➢ Put the contents of the bowl with the marinade in a pan and cook for 3 minutes.
- ➢ Now add the tempeh cubes and cook until the outside of it is golden brown.
- ➢ Season with salt and pepper, stir one last time and turn off.
- ➢ Put the tempeh on serving plates, sprinkle with the cooking juices and serve.

Nuts and berries crumble

Servings: 4 I Prep time: 10 minutes I Cook time: 15 minutes
Nutrition facts per serving: calories: 260; carbs 7.8 gr; protein 9 gr; fat 14 gr.

Ingredients
- ✓ 80 gr of almond flour

✓ 50 gr of mix nuts (walnuts, hazelnuts, pistachios)
✓ 200 gr of berries
✓ 20 ml of dissolved coconut oil
✓ 240 gr of soy yogurt

Directions
➢ Start by preheating the oven to 200° c.
➢ Then peel and chop all dried fruits.
➢ In a fairly large bowl, combine the almond flour, a pinch of stevia, the coconut oil, the chopped nuts and a pinch of salt.
➢ Mix the ingredients with your hands until many grains have formed.
➢ Pour the mixture into a baking tray covered with parchment paper and cook for 12 minutes, stirring the mixture from time to time to prevent it from burning.
➢ In the meantime, move on to preparing the cake bases.
➢ Wash and dry berries, remove the stalk, and then cut into small pieces.
➢ Put 60 gr of soy yogurt and 50 gr of berries in each of the 4 glasses you have prepared.
➢ After that put them in the fridge to rest.
➢ When the nuts crumble is cooked, remove it from the oven and let it cool.
➢ As soon as it is cold, take the glasses with the berries and yogurt from the fridge and sprinkle them with the grains and then serve.

Olives and tomato tofu

Servings: 4 I Prep time: 10 minutes I Cook time: 5 minutes
Nutrition facts per serving: calories: 190; carbs 5 gr; protein 11 gr; fat 6 gr.

Ingredients
✓ 400 gr of tofu
✓ 200 gr of cherry tomatoes
✓ 100 gr of green olives
✓ 1 teaspoon of dried oregano

Directions
➢ Rinse and pat the seitan with a paper towel and then cut it into strips.
➢ Wash the cherry tomatoes and then cut them into four wedges.
➢ Heat two tablespoons of oil in a pan and as soon as it is hot, add the cherry tomatoes.
➢ Sauté them for two minutes and then add the seitan slices.
➢ Cook for 3 minutes. Season with salt and pepper, mix and finally add the pitted green olives.
➢ Continue cooking for another two minutes. Turn off and sprinkle everything with

oregano.
➢ Now put the seitan and the vegetables on serving dishes.
➢ You can serve.

Orange and basil tofu

Servings: 4 I Prep time: 10 minutes I Cook time: 10 minutes
Nutrition facts per serving: calories: 160; carbs 6 gr; protein 14 gr; fat 2 gr.

Ingredients
✓ 600 gr of tofu
✓ 6 basil leaves
✓ 1 orange
✓ 30 gr of soy butter
✓ 2 tbsp of soy flour

Directions
➢ First, rinse the seitan and pat it dry with absorbent paper, then cut it into slices.
➢ Put 2 tbsp soy flour on a plate and flour the slices of seitan.
➢ Wash and chop basil leaves.
➢ Wash the orange, remove the zest, and strain the juice into a bowl.
➢ Put the butter in a pan and as soon as it has melted, add the chopped basil leaves and orange zest.
➢ Toast for a couple of minutes, and then add the slices of seitan.
➢ Brown them for 2 minutes on each side and then add salt, pepper, and orange juice.
➢ Continue cooking for another 5 minutes and then turn off.
➢ Put the slices on serving plates, sprinkle them with the cooking juices and serve.

Raspberry and soy mousse

Servings: 4 I Prep time: 10 minutes + 1 hour in the fridgel Cook time: -
Nutrition facts per serving: calories: 140; carbs 8 gr; protein 6 gr; fat 4 gr.

Ingredients
✓ 200 gr of raspberries
✓ 20 gr of natural powdered stevia
✓ 380 ml of soy milk whipped cream
✓ 20 ml of soy milk
✓ 4 gr of agar agar powder

Directions

➢ First wash and clean the raspberries, and blend them with an immersion blender, until the mixture is smooth.
➢ Add agar agar powder and soy milk to the strawberry mixture and stir to mix.
➢ Whip the soymilk cream and stevia, with an electric mixer in a clean bowl and incorporate it several times, stirring from the bottom up, to the raspberry mixture.
➢ When you have obtained a homogeneous mixture, divide it into the chosen glasses.
➢ Refrigerate for 1 hour before serving.
➢ After this time, you can serve your raspberries and soy mousse.

Rocket seeds and cucumber salad

Servings: 4 I Prep time: 10 minutes I Cook time: -
Nutrition facts per serving: calories: 90; carbs 4 gr; protein 2 gr; fat 5 gr.

Ingredients
✓ 100 gr of rocket salad
✓ 1 small cucumber
✓ 2 tablespoons of sesame seeds
✓ 1 teaspoon of chia seeds
✓ Olive oil, salt and pepper to taste

Directions
➢ First, clean and wash the rocket salad.
➢ Meanwhile, peel, wash and cut the cucumber into slices.
➢ Combine the cucumber slices, the rocket salad, chia seeds and the sesame seeds in a bowl or serving dish.
➢ Season with the olive oil, salt and pepper and mix well before serving.
➢ Serve your salad.

Soy cheese and peppers

Servings: 4 I Prep time: 10 minutes I Cook time: 10 minutes
Nutrition facts per serving: calories: 180; carbs 7.8 gr; protein 10 gr; fat 3 gr.

Ingredients
✓ ½ red bell pepper
✓ 20 green olives
✓ 3 tablespoons of pickled capers
✓ 200 gr of soy cheese
✓ Olive oil to taste

Directions
➢ First clean pepper, removing the stalk, then wash it.

➢ Let grill the bell peppers cut lengthwise into four pieces on a plate.
➢ Let them cool for about ten minutes and then remove the peel.
➢ Meanwhile, chop the olives and capers.
➢ Combine them with soy cheese in a pan.
➢ Mix well all ingredients.
➢ Arrange the peppers in a pan, sprinkle with the soy cheese and add a drizzle of oil.
➢ They can be served cold or at room temperature.

Soy cheese and cocoa dessert

Servings: 4 I Prep time: 10 minutes I Cook time: -
Nutrition facts per serving: calories: 210; carbs 9 gr; protein 8 gr; fat 6 gr.

Ingredients
✓ 200 gr of soy cheese
✓ 50 gr of unsweetened cocoa powder
✓ 10 ml of natural liquid stevia
✓ 200 ml of soymilk whipping cream
✓ 1 teaspoon of vanilla extract

Directions
➢ First, take a bowl and put the soy cheese inside.
➢ With an electric mixer, start working the cheese until you have obtained a light and fluffy cream.
➢ Set the mixer to minimum speed and add the vanilla extract first and then the soy cream.
➢ While continuing to mix, add the stevia and stir until well blended.
➢ Now, add the cocoa powder and a pinch of salt, increase the speed of the mixer to the maximum and continue to mix for another 2 minutes, or in any case until you have obtained a soft and homogeneous mixture.
➢ Put the mousse to rest in the fridge for an hour and then serve it in four glasses.

Soy aubergine

Servings: 4 I Prep time: 15 minutes I Cook time: 20 minutes
Nutrition facts per serving: calories: 150; carbs 5.8 gr; protein 6 gr; fat 3 gr.

Ingredients
✓ 1 aubergine
✓ 30 ml of olive oil
✓ 40 gr of soy flour
✓ 15 gr of soy flours
✓ 1 tbsp of chopped parsley
✓ Olive oil and salt

Directions

- First, soak aubergine with water and salt for at least 10 minute.
- After that time, rinse it under running water.
- Then cut it into slices, but not too thinly.
- Brush with olive oil into a bowl, distributing it over the entire surface.
- Then lay down the aubergine slices, being careful to overlap each other.
- Meanwhile, preheat the oven to 200° c.
- Mix the soy flour with the breadcrumbs on a plate.
- Add a pinch of salt, pepper, a little of washed and chopped parsley.
- Stir again to mix your breading.
- Arrange the mixture thus obtained on the zucchini, trying to distribute it evenly.
- Add the other tablespoon of oil over the aubergine and cook for about 20 minutes, or in any case, until golden brown.
- Take out of the oven and serve after letting it cool for a few minutes.
- You can serve your soy aubergine.

Spinach and ginger cream

Servings: 4 I Prep time: 10 minutes I Cook time: 20 minutes
Nutrition facts per serving: calories: 60; carbs 3 gr; protein 8 gr; fat 1 gr.

Ingredients
- ✓ 300 gr of spinach leaves
- ✓ 1 white onion
- ✓ 1 tsp of chopped fresh ginger
- ✓ Olive oil to taste, salt and pepper

Directions
- First peel and wash the onion then chop it.
- Wash and grate 1 tsp of fresh ginger.
- Rinse the spinach leaves under running water and then let them drain.
- Put a tablespoon of olive oil in a saucepan and as soon as it is hot, put the onion to fry for a couple of minutes.
- Now add the spinach and ginger.
- Mix all ingredients and season with salt and pepper.
- Now add 300 ml of water and cook for 20 minutes.
- After 20 minutes, take half of the spinach and set them aside.
- Blend the rest with an immersion blender until you get a smooth and creamy mixture.
- Put the cream on the plates, season it with a drizzle of olive oil and serve.

Strawberry and stevia mousse

Servings: 4 I Prep time: 10 minutes I Cook time: 30 minutes
Nutrition facts per serving: calories: 130; carbs 8 gr; protein 2 gr; fat 5 gr.

Ingredients
- ✓ 250 gr of strawberries
- ✓ 20 gr of natural stevia
- ✓ 400 ml of soy milk whipped cream
- ✓ 4 gr of agar agar powder
- ✓ 10-12 fresh strawberries for decoration

Directions
- First wash the strawberries, removing the stalk, and blend them with an immersion blender, until the mixture is smooth.
- Add agar agar powder to the strawberry mixture and stir to mix.
- In a clean dish, whip the soymilk cream and stevia with an electric mixer until smooth, then fold it into the strawberry mixture several times, swirling from the bottom up.
- When you have obtained a homogeneous mixture, divide it into the chosen glasses.
- Refrigerate for 1 hour before serving.
- Once you have a homogenous mixture, divide it into the glasses of your choice.

Thyme and courgettes stuffed tomatoes

Servings: 4 I Prep time: 10 minutes I Cook time: 10 minutes + 30 minutes of rest in the fridge
Nutrition facts per serving: calories: 115; carbs 7.8 gr; protein 12 gr; fat 4 gr.

Ingredients
- ✓ 10 piccadilly tomatoes
- ✓ 1 zucchini
- ✓ 1 tsp of chopped thyme
- ✓ 1 tsp of smoked paprika
- ✓ 2 tbsp extra virgin olive oil and salt

Directions
- First, wash the tomatoes, cut off the top and with a teaspoon, empty them of seeds.
- Let them drain upside down and in the meantime move on to preparing the filling.
- Peel and cut the courgette into very small pieces.
- Sauté them in a non-stick pan with a drizzle of oil for about ten minutes, adding paprika and salt.
- Fill the tomatoes with the courgette, using a teaspoon.

- ➢ Leave them to flavour in the fridge for at least 30 minutes.
- ➢ You can serve.

Tofu and basil aubergine

Servings: 4 I Prep time: 10 minutes I Cook time: 20 minutes
Nutrition facts per serving: calories: 160; carbs 8.8 gr; protein 14 gr; fat 5 gr.

Ingredients
- ✓ 1 aubergine
- ✓ 2 tbsp of olive oil
- ✓ 40 gr of almond flour
- ✓ 15 gr of grated tofu
- ✓ 1 tbsp of chopped basil

Directions
- ➢ Start by soaking aubergine with water and salt for at least 10 minute.
- ➢ After that time, rinse it under running water.
- ➢ Then cut it into slices, but not too thinly.
- ➢ Brush with olive oil into a bowl, distributing it over the entire surface.
- ➢ Then lay down the aubergine slices, being careful to overlap each other.
- ➢ Meanwhile, preheat the oven to 200° c.
- ➢ Mix the almond flour with grated tofu on a plate.
- ➢ Add a pinch of salt, pepper, a little of washed and chopped basil.
- ➢ Stir again to mix your tofu breading.
- ➢ Arrange the mixture thus obtained on the zucchini, trying to distribute it evenly.
- ➢ Add the other tablespoon of oil over the aubergine and cook for about 20 minutes, or in any case, until golden brown.
- ➢ Take out of the oven and serve after letting it cool for a few minutes.
- ➢ You can serve.

Tofu and soy biscuits

Servings: 4 I Prep time: 10 minutes I Cook time: 10 minutes
Nutrition facts per serving: calories: 215; carbs 7.8 gr; protein 21 gr; fat 5 gr.

Ingredients
- ✓ 40 gr grated tofu cheese
- ✓ 100 gr of soy flour
- ✓ 1 teaspoon baking soda
- ✓ 40 gr of soy butter
- ✓ 60 ml of soy milk
- ✓ Olive oil, backing powder and salt

Directions
- ➢ In a large bowl, mix the soy flour, baking soda, and salt.
- ➢ Use your fingers or a pastry cutter to work the cubed butter into the flour until the pieces are pea sized.
- ➢ Add the tofu cheese and onion and keep melting to mix all ingredients.
- ➢ Add the soy milk too.
- ➢ Stir until the milk and flour come together to form a dough.
- ➢ Flour should be lightly dusted over the work surface. Place the dough on a work surface.
- ➢ Press the dough with your hands into a 12-inch-thick, 8-inch-diameter disk. Using a lightly floured 2 1/2-inch round cutter, cut out six rounds of dough. When you get to number ten, make sure you press straight down. Cutting the dough is necessary because twisting it will prevent it from rising.
- ➢ Lightly brush the baking pan with a bit of olive oil.
- ➢ Then, arrange the biscuits in a single layer on the baking pan.
- ➢ Place the pan in the oven at 200°c.
- ➢ Let biscuits cooking for about to 10 minutes or cook until the biscuits are golden brown.
- ➢ When biscuits will be done, serve still hot.

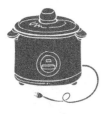

Slow cooker recipes

In this special section we want to provide you with 51 additional recipes to be made in the slow cooker.
They are always low-carb recipes, with a maximum of 5 ingredients, divided into specific categories.

Breakfast slow cooker recipes

Almond and berries cobbler

Servings: 4 I Prep time: 10 minutes I Cook time: 2 hours
Nutrition facts per serving: calories: 270; carbs: 9 gr; protein: 13 gr; fat: 10 gr.

Ingredients
- ✓ 200 gr of almond flour
- ✓ 30 gr of stevia
- ✓ 200 ml of almond milk
- ✓ 1 tbsp of vanilla powder
- ✓ About 400 gr of berries
- ✓ Backing powder

Directions
- ➢ First, wash, dry and cut the berries into small pieces.
- ➢ Put almond flour, stevia, 1 tsp of baking soda in a bowl and mix together the dry ingredients.
- ➢ Add the milk a little at a time, until you get a smooth batter.
- ➢ Now, take another little butter and grease the slow cooker generously.
- ➢ Put the berries on the bottom and cover them with the dough.
- ➢ Place a cloth (or a layer of paper towel) under the lid to absorb the moisture and cook for 2 hours in high mode.
- ➢ You can serve your cobbler with low-carb ice cream.

Bacon and cheddar savoury pie

Servings: 4 I Prep time: 10 minutes I Cook time: 2 hours and 30 minutes
Nutrition facts per serving: calories: 290; carbs: 9 gr; protein: 13 gr; fat: 14 gr.

Ingredients
- ✓ 400 gr of almond flour
- ✓ 300 ml of unsweetened almond milk
- ✓ 2 eggs
- ✓ 100 g of sliced bacon
- ✓ 60 gr of grated cheddar cheese
- ✓ Instant yeast
- ✓ Salt and pepper

Directions
- ➢ First, cut the bacon into fairly thick strips.
- ➢ Meanwhile, put the flour with almond milk in a bowl.
- ➢ Beat the eggs and add them to the previously made mixture.
- ➢ Mix everything with the help of a whisk for a few minutes, adding a spoonful of instant yeast until the dough is compact.
- ➢ Insert the bacon, and grated cheddar cheese, and pepper.
- ➢ Let the mixture rest for 5 minutes so that it begins to rise which will then continue during cooking.
- ➢ Switch on cooking the savoury pie in the slow cooker.
- ➢ Grease the slow cooker pan and pour the mixture inside.
- ➢ Set the high mode and cook for 2 and a half hours (however, check the progress of cooking with a toothpick).
- ➢ Once cooked, allow the cake to cool before cutting it into slices and serving it for breakfast.

Blueberry and coconut pancake

Servings: 4 I Prep time: 10 minutes I Cook time: 2 hours
Nutrition facts per serving: calories: 190; carbs: 9 gr; protein: 8 gr; fat: 8 gr.

Ingredients
- ✓ 200 gr coconut flour
- ✓ 200 gr of blueberries
- ✓ 2 eggs
- ✓ 120 ml coconut milk
- ✓ 1 tsp of baking powder + salt

Directions
- ➢ First, mix coconut flour, 1 tsp of baking powder, a pinch of baking soda and salt in medium bowl.
- ➢ Meanwhile, wash and dry blueberries.
- ➢ In a large bowl add coconut milk, eggs and whisk together.

➤ Slowly combine the dry and wet ingredients, stirring constantly, until no lumps remain.
➤ Fold in the blueberries carefully.
➤ Spray the crock liberally with nonstick cooking spray.
➤ Cook on high for 2 hours, or until the edges are lightly browned and the centre is thoroughly cooked.
➤ Allow to cool for 10 minutes uncovered before slicing and serving your pancake with a sprinkle of coconut flour.

Brie and speck breakfast little soy pie

Servings: 4 I Prep time: 10 minutes I Cook time: 2 hours and 30 minutes
Nutrition facts per serving: calories: 230; carbs: 10.8 gr; protein: 16 gr; fat: 6 gr.

Ingredients
✓ 300 gr of soy flour
✓ 300 ml of unsweetened soy milk
✓ 2 eggs
✓ 100 gr of diced speck
✓ 60 gr of brie
✓ Olive oil

Directions
➤ First, cut the speck into little slices.
➤ Meanwhile, put the soy flour with soy milk and 20 ml of olive oil in a bowl.
➤ Beat the eggs and add them to the previously made mixture.
➤ Mix everything with the help of a whisk for a few minutes, adding a spoonful of instant yeast until the dough is compact.
➤ Insert the speck brie.
➤ Grease the slow cooker pan and pour the mixture inside.
➤ Set the high mode and cook for 2 and a half hours (always check the progress of cooking with a toothpick).
➤ Once cooked, allow the cake to cool before cutting it into slices and serving it for breakfast.

Cinnamon and soy crumble pie

Servings: 4 I Prep time: 10 minutes I Cook time: 2 hours
Nutrition facts per serving: calories: 200; carbs: 7 gr; protein: 14 gr; fat: 7 gr.

Ingredients
✓ 200 gr of soy flour
✓ 40 gr of stevia

✓ 200 ml of soy milk
✓ 1 tbsp of cinnamon powder
✓ 4 tbsp of chopped hazelnuts
✓ Backing powder

Directions
➤ First, finely chop hazelnuts.
➤ Put soy flour, stevia, 1 tsp of baking soda in a bowl and mix together the dry ingredients.
➤ Add the milk a little at a time, until you get a smooth batter.
➤ Add the cinnamon powder.
➤ Now, take another little olive oil and grease the slow cooker generously.
➤ Put the hazelnuts on the bottom and cover them with the dough.
➤ Place a cloth (or a layer of paper towel) under the lid to absorb the moisture and cook for 2 hours in high mode.
➤ Allow to cool and serve your crumble pie for breakfast.

Cinnamon rolls

Servings: 4 I Prep time: 10 minutes I Cook time: 2 hours
Nutrition facts per serving: calories: 180; carbs: 9 gr; protein: 9 gr; fat: 6 gr.

Ingredients
✓ 300 gr of almond flour
✓ 40 gr of butter
✓ 40 gr of stevia powder (10 for the dough and 30 for the filling)
✓ 1 egg
✓ 10 gr of cinnamon powder
✓ Instant yeast

Directions
➤ First, melt the butter in the microwave or in a saucepan in a double boiler and then let it come to room temperature.
➤ Meanwhile, in a bowl, mix 10 gr of stevia, almond flour, and 10 gr dry yeast.
➤ In another container, mix the egg and 100 ml of water at room temperature.
➤ Combine the three parts and knead the dough with your hands. After obtaining a ball, let it rise at room temperature (about 25 °) for an hour covered with cling film. After this time, roll out the dough with a rolling pin giving it a rectangular shape.
➤ Finally brush over with melted butter.
➤ Prepare a mix of stevia and cinnamon and sprinkle over the dough already spread evenly.

- ➢ Roll the dough on itself forming a kind of sausage and then cut into thick enough slices starting from the centre as is done for sushi.
- ➢ Cook for 2 hours on high mode.
- ➢ Place a cloth between the pan and the lid to absorb any condensation that forms during cooking.
- ➢ When cooked, remove the cinnamon rolls from the slow cooker by lifting them directly with the parchment paper and allow to cool for a few minutes.
- ➢ You can serve your rolls.

Coconut and cinnamon rolls

Servings: 4 I Prep time: 10 minutes I Cook time: 2 hours
Nutrition facts per serving: calories: 160; carbs: 12.8 gr; protein: 12 gr; fat: 6 gr.

Ingredients
- ✓ 300 gr of coconut flour
- ✓ 4 tbsp of coconut oil
- ✓ 50 gr of stevia powder (20 for the dough and 30 for the filling)
- ✓ 1 egg
- ✓ 10 gr of cinnamon powder

Directions
- ➢ First, melt the coconut oil in the microwave or in a saucepan in a double boiler and then let it come to room temperature.
- ➢ Meanwhile, in a bowl, mix 10 gr of stevia, coconut flour, 1 tsp of baking powder and a pinch of salt.
- ➢ In another container, mix the egg, 60 ml of coconut milk and 60 ml of water at room temperature.
- ➢ Combine the three parts and knead the dough with your hands.
- ➢ After obtaining a ball, let it rise at room temperature (about 25 °) for an hour covered with cling film. After this time, roll out the dough with a rolling pin giving it a rectangular shape.
- ➢ Finally brush over with melted coconut oil.
- ➢ Prepare a mix of stevia and cinnamon and sprinkle over the dough already spread evenly.
- ➢ Roll the dough on itself forming a kind of sausage and then cut into thick enough slices starting from the centre as is done for sushi. For the 3-liter slow cooker 6 swivels are enough, while for the 6-liter one it takes about ten.
- ➢ Wet a sheet of baking paper and place it in the pot, then lay the swivels quite far from each other inside.

- ➢ Sprinkle everything with more sugar and cook for 2 hours on high mode.
- ➢ Place a cloth between the pan and the lid to absorb any condensation that forms during cooking.
- ➢ When cooked, remove the rolls from the slow cooker by lifting them directly with the parchment paper and allow to cool for a few minutes.
- ➢ You can serve your coconut and cinnamon rolls.

Easy omelette

Servings: 4 I Prep time: 10 minutes I Cook time: 40 minutes
Nutrition facts per serving: calories: 120; carbs: 2 gr; protein: 9 gr; fat: 7 gr.

Ingredients
- ✓ 6 eggs
- ✓ 30 ml of skimmed milk
- ✓ 2 tbsp of butter

Directions
- ➢ First, break the eggs into a bowl and pour in the milk. Skip it.
- ➢ Using a whisk, swirl the mixture until the first bubbles appear.
- ➢ Grease the bottom and sides of the slow cooker bowl with oil and pour the egg-milk mixture into them.
- ➢ Close the lid and install the cooking program. Cook for 20 minutes.
- ➢ After 5 minutes, remove the lid.
- ➢ Remove the omelette from the bowl and set it on a prepared flat dish.
- ➢ This must be done to prevent the omelette from falling out because to the temperature differential.
- ➢ Cook the other side for other 10/15 minutes.
- ➢ Once is ready you can serve your omelette still hot.

Nut breakfast pie

Servings: 4 I Prep time: 10 minutes I Cook time: 2 hours
Nutrition facts per serving: calories: 190; carbs: 4 gr; protein: 9 gr; fat: 8 gr.

Ingredients
- ✓ 200 gr of almond flour
- ✓ 6 tbsp of chopped pistachios and walnuts
- ✓ 30 gr of stevia
- ✓ 200 ml of almond milk
- ✓ 1 tbsp of almond flavour

✓ Backing soda
Directions
➢ First, wash, take pistachios and walnuts and chop 6 tbsp of them.
➢ Put almond flour, chopped nuts stevia, 1 tsp of baking soda in a bowl and mix together.
➢ Melt 50 gr of butter and add it to the bowl.
➢ You will get a crumbled dough to which you add the almond milk a little at a time, until you get a smooth batter.
➢ Add the almond flavour too.
➢ Now, take another little olive oil and grease the slow cooker generously.
➢ Put the strawberries on the bottom and cover them with the dough.
➢ Place a cloth (or a layer of paper towel) under the lid to absorb the moisture and cook for 2 hours in high mode.
➢ Allow to cool and serve your nuts and oat pie for breakfast.

Pistachio scone

Servings: 4 I Prep time: 10 minutes I Cook time: 2 hours
Nutrition facts per serving: calories: 290; carbs: 8 gr; protein: 13 gr; fat: 14 gr.

Ingredients
✓ 300 gr of almond flour
✓ 300 ml of unsweetened almond milk
✓ 2 eggs
✓ 4 tbsp of chopped pistachios
✓ 60 gr of grated parmesan cheese
✓ Instant yeast
Directions
➢ First, finely chop pistachios.
➢ Meanwhile, put the almond flour and milk.
➢ Beat the eggs and add them to the previously made mixture.
➢ Mix everything with the help of a whisk for a few minutes, adding a spoonful of instant yeast until the dough is compact.
➢ Insert the pistachios and parmesan.
➢ Let the mixture rest for 5 minutes so that it begins to rise which will then continue during cooking.
➢ Switch on cooking the savoury pie in the slow cooker.
➢ Grease the slow cooker pan and pour the mixture inside.
➢ Set the high mode and cook for 2 and a half hours (however, check the progress of cooking with a toothpick).
➢ Once cooked, allow the cake to cool before cutting it into slices and serving it for breakfast.

Raspberry and vanilla pancake

Servings: 4 I Prep time: 10 minutes I Cook time: 2 hours
Nutrition facts per serving: calories: 180; carbs: 8.8 gr; protein: 8 gr; fat: 6 gr.

Ingredients
✓ 300 gr almond flour
✓ 200 gr of raspberries
✓ 2 eggs
✓ 120 ml almond milk
✓ 1 tsp of vanilla extract
✓ Backing soda + salt
Directions
➢ First, mix flour, 2 tsp of stevia, a pinch of baking soda and salt in medium bowl.
➢ Meanwhile, wash and dry raspberries, then cut into pieces.
➢ In a large bowl add almond milk, eggs and whisk together.
➢ Slowly add dry mixture to wet ingredients and stir until no lumps remain.
➢ Carefully fold the prepared mix in raspberries, careful not to stir very much.
➢ Spray crock very well with non-stick spray.
➢ Pour batter into the pot and cover.
➢ Cook on high slow cooker function, for 2 hours until edges are slightly browned, and the centre is fully cooked through.
➢ Let cool uncovered for 10 minutes then slice your pancake and serve.

Parmesan scone

Servings: 4 I Prep time: 10 minutes I Cook time: 2 hours and 30 minutes
Nutrition facts per serving: calories: 240; carbs: 8 gr; protein: 11 gr; fat: 5 gr.

Ingredients
✓ 300 gr of almond flour
✓ 300 ml of unsweetened almond milk
✓ 2 eggs
✓ 100 gr of cooked ham (diced)
✓ 60 g parmesan cheese (grated)
✓ Instant yeast
Directions
➢ First, cut the cooked ham into fairly thick cubes.
➢ Meanwhile, put the flour with milk and 20 ml of olive oil in a bowl.
➢ Beat the eggs and add them to the previously made mixture.

- Mix everything with the help of a whisk for a few minutes, adding a spoonful of instant yeast until the dough is compact.
- Insert the cooked ham, cheese, and pepper.
- Let the mixture "breathe" for 5 minutes so that it begins to rise which will then continue during cooking.
- Switch on cooking the savoury pie in the slow cooker.
- Grease the slow cooker pan and pour the mixture inside.
- Set the high mode and cook for 2 and a half hours (however, check the progress of cooking with a toothpick).
- Once cooked, allow the cake to cool before cutting it into slices and serving it for breakfast.

Strawberry pie

Servings: 4 | Prep time: 10 minutes | Cook time: 2 hours
Nutrition facts per serving: calories: 160; carbs: 8 gr; protein: 7 gr; fat: 8 gr.

Ingredients
- ✓ 200 gr of almond flour
- ✓ 300 gr of strawberries
- ✓ 30 gr of stevia
- ✓ 200 ml of coconut milk
- ✓ 1 tbsp of vanilla powder
- ✓ Backing soda + salt

Directions
- First, wash, dry and cut the strawberries into small pieces.
- Put almond flour, stevia, 1 tsp of baking soda + 1 pinch of salt in a bowl and mix together.
- Add the coconut milk a little at a time, until you get a smooth batter.
- Add the vanilla powder.
- Now, take another little olive oil and grease the slow cooker generously.
- Put the strawberries on the bottom and cover them with the dough.
- Place a cloth (or a layer of paper towel) under the lid to absorb the moisture and cook for 2 hours in high mode.
- Allow to cool and serve your pie for breakfast.

Vanilla rolls

Servings: 4 | Prep time: 10 minutes | Cook time: 2 hours
Nutrition facts per serving: calories: 190; carbs: 9 gr; protein: 8 gr; fat: 6 gr.

Ingredients
- ✓ 300 gr of almond flour
- ✓ 60 ml of almond milk
- ✓ 50 gr of stevia powder (20 for the dough and 30 for the filling)
- ✓ 1 egg
- ✓ 10 gr of vanilla powder
- ✓ Backing soda + salt

Directions
- First, in a bowl, mix 10 gr of stevia, oat flour, 1 tsp of baking soda and a pinch of salt.
- In another container, mix the egg, 60 ml of almond milk and 60 ml of water at room temperature.
- Combine the three parts and knead the dough with your hands.
- After obtaining a ball, let it rise at room temperature (about 25 °) for an hour covered with cling film. After this time, roll out the dough with a rolling pin giving it a rectangular shape.
- Finally brush over with a bit of olive oil.
- Prepare a mix of stevia and vanilla and sprinkle over the dough already spread evenly.
- Roll the dough on itself forming a kind of sausage and then cut into thick enough slices starting from the centre as is done for sushi.
- Wet a sheet of baking paper and place it in the pot, then lay the swivels quite far from each other inside.
- Cook for 2 hours on high mode.
- Place a cloth between the pan and the lid to absorb any condensation that forms during cooking.
- When cooked, remove the vanilla rolls from the slow cooker by lifting them directly with the parchment paper and allow to cool for a few minutes.
- You can serve your rolls for breakfast.

Walnut pancake

Servings: 4 | Prep time: 10 minutes | Cook time: 2 hours
Nutrition facts per serving: calories: 200; carbs: 6 gr; protein: 9 gr; fat: 12 gr.

Ingredients
- ✓ 300 gr almond flour
- ✓ 4 tbsp of chopped walnuts
- ✓ 2 eggs
- ✓ 120 ml almond milk
- ✓ Stevia
- ✓ 1 tsp of baking soda + salt

Directions

- First, mix almond flour, 2 tsp of stevia, 2 tsp of baking soda and salt in medium bowl.
- Meanwhile, finely chop walnuts (leaving 1 tbsp aside).
- In a large bowl add oat milk, eggs and whisk together.
- Slowly add dry mixture to wet ingredients and stir until no lumps remain.
- Carefully fold the prepared mix in 3 tbsp of chopped walnuts, careful not to stir very much.
- Spray crock very well with non-stick spray.
- Pour batter into crock and cover your slow cooker.
- Cook on high slow cooker function, for 2 hours until edges are slightly browned, and the centre is fully cooked through.
- Let cool uncovered for 10 minutes then slice your pancake and serve with a sprinkle of remaining walnuts.

Meat slow cooker recipes

Artichokes and bacon pork loin

Servings: 4 I Prep time: 10 minutes I Cook time: 1/2 hours
Nutrition facts per serving: calories: 390; carbs: 6 gr; protein: 34 gr; fat: 12 gr.

Ingredients
- 1 kg of pork loin
- 100 gr of bacon
- 3 artichokes
- 1 tbsp of mixed spices

Directions
- First, wash and dry the pork loin. With a very sharp knife, cut the loin so that it can then be rolled up.
- Once opened, put the bacon and spices inside.
- Roll everything up and with a wire for roasts tie the loin so that it is very compact.
- At this point, cut and clean the artichokes, first putting them in a bowl of water and vinegar to prevent them from turning black.
- Arrange the pork loin at the bottom of the pot, then add the artichokes as well.
- Cook for 5 hours at low, if you have a probe thermometer, set it to a core temperature of around 75/80 degrees.
- Once cooked, put it in warm and always let it rest inside the slow cooker for about 1 or 2 hours.

- At the end take out the loin, if you want you can quickly pass it in a pan to make the surface nice crunchy.
- You can cut it and serve it on the serving plates surrounded by artichokes.

Aubergine and spices chicken legs

Servings: 4 I Prep time: 10 minutes I Cook time: 5 hours
Nutrition facts per serving: calories: 390; carbs: 6 gr; protein: 34 gr; fat: 12 gr.

Ingredients
- 6 chicken legs
- 2 aubergines
- 1 tbsp of powder garlic
- 1tbsp of powder onion
- salt

Directions
- First, peel the aubergines, wash them, and cut them lengthwise, they must become wide and low.
- Put on the bottom of the pot, they will serve as a rise.
- Then, wash and season the chicken legs with salt, pepper, oil, garlic, and onion powder.
- Place them in the slow cooker pot and turn on to low mode.
- Cooking must last 5 hours.
- After the time has elapsed, turn on the grill of the oven and put the chicken legs and potatoes in a baking dish, pass a little more oil, then let them toast for 10 minutes.
- Once they are golden on the surface, remove them from the oven and serve.
- Serve chicken legs surrounded by aubergines and with cooking juices.

Aubergine roasted veal

Servings: 4 I Prep time: 10 minutes I Cook time: 4 hours
Nutrition facts per serving: calories: 420; carbs: 7 gr; protein: 34 gr; fat: 6 gr.

Ingredients
- 1 kg of lean roast veal
- 250 ml of meat broth
- 2 aubergines
- 2 cloves of garlic
- Olive oil, salt and pepper

Directions

- First, wash and peel both the aubergines and chop them coarsely.
- Wash, dry and season the meat with salt and pepper.
- Peel wash and mince garlic cloves.
- Pour two tablespoons of oil into a pan, preferably cast iron, and sear the roast on each side for a few minutes.
- Blanch the aubergines, carrots, and crushed garlic in the still hot pan for 5 minutes.
- Now switch to cooking the veal roast in the slow cooker.
- Place the roast in the slow cooker.
- Pour the vegetables around the roast inside the slow cooker.
- Add the marjoram (or thyme if you prefer) and cover with the broth.
- Turn the slow cooker on high for 4 hours.
- Once cooking is complete, remove the roast from the pan and remove any net or wire that may be present, slice as desired and place in a bowl together with the vegetables removed from the pot, preserving the remaining liquid.
- The ideal accompaniment for roasts is a cream made with the cooking liquid and a spoonful of corn-starch, to be reduced in a saucepan for a few minutes, to be poured over the meat and vegetables.
- You can serve your veal dish.

Coconut milk and rosemary pork loin

Servings: 4 I Prep time: 10 minutes I Cook time: 5 hours
Nutrition facts per serving: calories: 310; carbs: 2 gr; protein: 32 gr; fat: 7gr.

Ingredients
- ✓ 850 gr of pork loin
- ✓ 300 ml of unsweetened coconut milk
- ✓ 2 tbsp of chopped red onion
- ✓ 1 sprig of rosemary
- ✓ Olive oil, salt and pepper

Directions
- First, take the pork loin, wash it, and dry it with a paper towel.
- Wash and chop 2 tablespoons of red onion.
- Wash and chop the rosemary too.
- Place the meat in the pot and pour the coconut milk over it.
- Add the onion, rosemary, salt, pepper, and a drop of olive oil.
- Now you can turn on the slow cooker and enter the low mode and let it cook for 5 hours.

- When cooked, separate the piece of meat, and let it cool for a few minutes wrapped in aluminium foil.
- When it is almost at room temperature it will be ready and very soft to be sliced.
- In the meantime, collect the cooking liquids with the onion and use a mixer to blend everything and obtain a sauce to pour over the meat.
- Then use a saucepan to thicken until the desired result is obtained.
- Arrange the slices of pork loin with milk in a baking dish and serve at the table.

Courgette and sage beef

Servings: 4 I Prep time: 10 minutes I Cook time: 4 hours
Nutrition facts per serving: calories: 420; carbs: 8 gr; protein: 34gr; fat: 6 gr.

Ingredients
- ✓ 1 kg of lean roast veal
- ✓ 250 ml of meat broth
- ✓ 2 courgettes
- ✓ 1 tbsp of finely chopped sage
- ✓ 2 garlic cloves
- ✓ Olive oil, salt and pepper

Directions
- First, wash and peel courgettes, and chop them coarsely.
- Wash and chop sage too.
- Wash, dry and season the meat with salt and pepper.
- Peel wash and mince garlic cloves.
- Pour two tablespoons of oil into a pan and sear the roast on each side for a few minutes.
- Blanch the courgettes, and crushed garlic in the still hot pan for 5 minutes.
- Now switch to cooking the veal roast in the slow cooker.
- Place the roast in the slow cooker.
- Pour the vegetables around the roast beef inside the slow cooker.
- Add the chopped sage and cover with the broth.
- Turn the slow cooker on high for 4 hours.
- Once cooking is complete, remove the roast from the pan and remove any net or wire that may be present, slice as desired and place in a bowl together with the vegetables removed from the pot, preserving the remaining liquid.
- You can serve your beef with cooking liquid and courgettes.

Curry and herbs pork stew

Servings: 4 I Prep time: 10 minutes I Cook time: 5 hours
Nutrition facts per serving: calories: 480; carbs: 3 gr; protein: 39 gr; fat: 18 gr.

Ingredients
- ✓ 1 kg of pork stew
- ✓ 2 tbsp of chopped mixed herbs
- ✓ 2 tsp of curry
- ✓ 2 tbsp of liquid stevia
- ✓ 2 tbsp of white wine
- ✓ Salt to taste

Directions
- ➤ First, create the emulsion for the meat.
- ➤ Combine the liquid ingredients first, then the stevia 2 tablespoons of olive oil and the wine. Mix the emulsion.
- ➤ Add the powdered spices and chopped aromatic herbs to the emulsion, mix well.
- ➤ Wash and remove excess fat from the pork.
- ➤ Wash and chop the garlic cloves.
- ➤ Put the stew in the slow cooker and pour over the spice emulsion, and the garlic cloves.
- ➤ Add salt to taste.
- ➤ Massage the meat with your hands to evenly distribute the seasoning.
- ➤ Now move on to cooking the pork with spices
- ➤ Cover and cook on high for 5 hours.
- ➤ After cooking, first remove the pieces of meat and set aside in a bowl.
- ➤ Let the meat rest, then cut it into small pieces and serve on serving plates.

Easy roast beef

Servings: 4 I Prep time: 10 minutes I Cook time:
Nutrition facts per serving: calories: 350; carbs: 2 gr; protein: 34 gr; fat: 6 gr.

Ingredients
- ✓ A cut of meat for a 1 kg roast beef
- ✓ 2 tbsp of red wine
- ✓ 2 tbsp of mixed spices

Directions
- ➤ First, roll the meat with a string so that it remains nice and compact, then massage with the spices.
- ➤ In a large pan, heat a little oil and then brown the meat on each side.
- ➤ At this point insert the thermometer trying to reach the centre of the piece of roast beef with the probe.
- ➤ Then put the meat in the slow cooker, and add the red wine to the pot, cover and turn on to low.

- ➤ Now you don't have to set a timer, but set an alarm temperature on the kitchen thermometer, remember that you will always have an increase of about 4/5 degrees after you have removed the meat from the pot.
- ➤ Then set the warning a few degrees lower than what you want to reach as the final temperature. Set the temperature to reach 58.
- ➤ When it reaches temperature, turn off the slow cooker, take out the roast beef and wrap it, together with the cooking liquids, inside the foil meat.
- ➤ Let it rest for a few hours, in a closed place rest is important to restore hydration to the meat.
- ➤ If you want, you can leave the probe still in the core to see what temperature it reaches.
- ➤ When it has cooled down, you just have to cut it into thin slices and serve it at the table.

Onion brandy and ginger pulled pork

Servings: 4 I Prep time: 10 minutes I Cook time: 5 hours
Nutrition facts per serving: calories: 480; carbs: 3 gr; protein: 39 gr; fat: 18 gr.

Ingredients
- ✓ 1 kg of pork stew
- ✓ 1 tbsp of powdered ginger
- ✓ 1 chopped red onion
- ✓ 2 tbsp of liquid stevia
- ✓ 2 tbsp of brandy
- ✓ Salt and pepper

Directions
- ➤ First, prepare the ginger and brandy marinade for the pork meat.
- ➤ Combine the liquid ingredients first, then the stevia, 2 tablespoons of olive oil and brandy.
- ➤ Mix the emulsion.
- ➤ Add the powdered ginger to the emulsion, mix well.
- ➤ Wash and remove excess fat from the pork.
- ➤ Wash and chop the red onion.
- ➤ Put the stew in the slow cooker and pour over the brandy and ginger marinade, and the chopped onion
- ➤ Add salt and pepper to taste.
- ➤ Massage the meat with your hands to evenly distribute the seasoning.
- ➤ Cover and cook on high for 5 hours.
- ➤ After cooking, first remove the pieces of meat.
- ➤ Shred the pork, set aside and season it with the cooking liquid, then serve.

Parmesan chicken wings

Servings: 4 I Prep time: 10 minutes I Cook time: 4 hours
Nutrition facts per serving: calories: 260; carbs: 3 gr; protein: 25 gr; fat: 8 gr.

Ingredients
- ✓ 900 gr of chicken wings
- ✓ 2 tbsp of minced garlic
- ✓ 1 cup of mayonnaise
- ✓ 4 tbsp of grated parmesan cheese
- ✓ 2 tsp of apple cider vinegar

Directions
- ➤ The first thing to do is to prepare the sauce.
- ➤ Peel, wash, and chop garlic.
- ➤ You need to mix all the ingredients together (mayonnaise, garlic, parmesan, and vinegar), except for the chicken wings, in a large bowl.
- ➤ Then go to grease the slow cooker pan with a little butter or using a special non-stick spray. Then pour half of the sauce over the bottom. Add the chicken wings and mix.
- ➤ Switch to cooking chicken wings with garlic and parmesan.
- ➤ Cook in the slow cooker with the lid on at maximum high temperature for 4 hours and then move to the preheated oven to make the fins crispier.
- ➤ Gently remove the wings from the slow cooker one at a time and arrange everything on a baking tray covered with aluminium foil. Pour the remaining sauce over the wings (spread the sauce well over the chicken with the help of a kitchen brush or a spoon) and cook in the oven with a grill for another 15 minutes at about 200 °c.
- ➤ Serve the chicken wings while still hot with a sprinkle of fresh parsley or basil and your favourite sauces.

Speck and oranges pork loin

Servings: 4 I Prep time: 10 minutes I Cook time: 6 hours
Nutrition facts per serving: calories: 360; carbs: 3 gr; protein: 34 gr; fat: 7 gr.

Ingredients
- ✓ 700 gr of pork loin in one piece
- ✓ 8 thick slices of speck
- ✓ 2 blood oranges
- ✓ 2 tbsp of liquid stevia
- ✓ Salt and pepper

Directions
- ➤ First, wash and dry the pork loin.
- ➤ Make incisions about one centimetre away in the pork loin, without reaching the end, opening it like a book.
- ➤ Wash and dry the oranges, then cut them into thin slices.
- ➤ Season with salt and pepper and insert, in each cut, a slice of speck and thin slices of orange.
- ➤ Pour over 2 tbsp of liquid stevia.
- ➤ Going gently from underneath, tie with kitchen twine to keep everything closed compactly.
- ➤ Butter, the slow cooker.
- ➤ Place the pork and turn on the slow cooker in low mode.
- ➤ Spend about 6 hours remove the meat from the pot and sprinkle the top and sides with honey. Finally, place on a baking sheet with parchment paper.
- ➤ Turn on the oven with the grill at maximum temperature and brown the loin with orange in the upper part of the oven for about 10 minutes.
- ➤ When it is well browned on the surface, remove from the oven, and let it rest for a few minutes before cutting and serving.
- ➤ You can serve your pork loin with the cooking liquid and orange slices.

Turkey nuggets with cheddar and broccoli

Servings: 4 I Prep time: 10 minutes I Cook time: 4 hours
Nutrition facts per serving: calories: 400; carbs: 4 gr; protein: 36 gr; fat: 10 gr.

Ingredients
- ✓ About 800 gr of turkey leg on the bone (or 500 boneless)
- ✓ 350 gr of clean broccoli flowers
- ✓ 2 tbsp of soy sauce
- ✓ 1 tsp of garlic powder
- ✓ 3 slices of cheddar cheese
- ✓ Salt and pepper

Directions
- ➤ First, wash the turkey and dry it.
- ➤ Slice the meat to obtain morsels, after removing the skin and any excess fat.
- ➤ Proceed to cut the vegetables: wash and slice a piece of onion and the broccoli flowers.
- ➤ Fry the onion in oil, if your slow cooker has the function for frying, or the inner pot can be placed on the stove, do it this way, otherwise fry in a separate pan and then move it to the slow cooker.

➢ When the onion begins to become transparent, add the garlic powder, and sauté for another 20 seconds.
➢ Then add the meat and let it sear for a couple of minutes.
➢ At this point you can start cooking in the slow cooker, then add the remaining ingredients: broccoli, soy sauce, salt, pepper and mix the ingredients.
➢ Set the pot to cook on high for 4 hours.
➢ after 4 hours, open the lid, if you notice that the liquid that has formed is excessive, you can leave the lid open for half an hour leaving it on high, or possibly set the frying function again if you have an instant pot, in so as to boil the liquid and reduce it.
➢ at this point, add the cheddar to the dish and wait for it to melt over the turkey bites.
➢ When it has melted you can distribute the turkey with broccoli directly on serving plates.
➢ You can serve.

Yogurt and mustard sauce chicken wings

Servings: 4 I Prep time: 10 minutes I Cook time: 4 hours
Nutrition facts per serving: calories: 280; carbs: 3 gr; protein: 29 gr; fat: 8 gr.

Ingredients
✓ 900 gr of chicken wings
✓ 2 tbsp of orange juice
✓ 200 gr of mayonnaise
✓ 100 gr of greek yogurt
✓ 1 tsp of chopped chives

Directions
➢ First, prepare yogurt and mustard sauce.
➢ Wash and chop chives.
➢ Now combine together in a bowl, mustard chives, orange juice and greek yogurt.
➢ Then go to grease the slow cooker pan with a little butter or using a special non-stick spray.
➢ Then pour half of the sauce over the bottom.
➢ Add the chicken wings and mix.
➢ Cook in the slow cooker with the lid on at maximum high temperature for 4 hours and then move to the preheated oven to make the fins crispier.
➢ Gently remove the wings from the slow cooker one at a time and arrange everything on a baking tray covered with aluminium foil.
➢ Pour the remaining sauce over the wings (spread the sauce well over the chicken with the help of a kitchen brush or a spoon) and cook in the oven with a grill for another 15 minutes at about 200 °c.
➢ Serve the chicken wings while still hot with a sprinkle of fresh parsley and the remaining sauce.

Fish slow cooker recipes

Aubergine and hake rolls

Servings: 4 I Prep time: 10 minutes I Cook time: 5 hours
Nutrition facts per serving: calories: 420; carbs: 12 gr; protein: 31 gr; fat: 6 gr.

Ingredients
✓ 400 gr of hake fillet
✓ 150 gr of tomato puree
✓ 2 aubergines
✓ 2 tbsp of italian pesto
✓ 8 black olives

Directions
➢ The first thing to do is wash and cut the aubergines into slices that are not too high, about half a centimetre thick.
➢ The cut must be made transversely in order to obtain the slices at their maximum length.
➢ Then move on to the hake fillets and cut them to the size of the aubergine slice.
➢ Place a little pesto on the fillet and wrap everything in the aubergine slice.
➢ With the help of a spoon, arrange the tomato puree and the olives previously cut into slices on top of the rolls.
➢ Once the rolls have been made, the preparation of the pot is started. It only takes a drizzle of oil on the bottom of the slow cooker and then the tomato puree left over from preparation must be added.
➢ Add salt and oregano and finally place the rolls inside the pot.
➢ Cook the rolls in high mode for 5 hours.
➢ Once the cook time is over, the rolls are ready to be served on the table.

Cuttelfish with feta and olives

Servings: 4 I Prep time: 10 minutes I Cook time: 4 hours
Nutrition facts per serving: calories: 460; carbs: 7 gr; protein: 42 gr; fat: 12 gr.

Ingredients
- ✓ 500 gr of clean cuttlefish
- ✓ 200 gr of greek feta
- ✓ 1 clove of garlic
- ✓ 100 gr of black olives
- ✓ 400 gr of peeled tomatoes

Directions
- ➢ First, peel and crush the garlic.
- ➢ Cut the feta into cubes about one centimetre.
- ➢ Wash and chop a little fresh parsley.
- ➢ Clean and let the cuttlefish dry.
- ➢ Fill the cuttlefish heads with feta, a little fresh parsley, and black olives.
- ➢ Now, fry the garlic in hot olive oil in a pan.
- ➢ When the garlic is golden, you can add the cuttlefish and fry them for a couple of minutes.
- ➢ Now you can move on to cooking cuttlefish with tomato in the slow cooker
- ➢ Put the oil in which we fried on the bottom of the slow cooker, add the cuttlefish, black olives, peeled tomatoes cut into pieces, oregano, salt, and pepper.
- ➢ Turn on the slow cooker by setting it to the highest high temperature, and let it cook for 4 hours.
- ➢ After 4 hours, turn off and serve the cuttlefish with tomato, olives, and feta.

Green olives and cherry tomato cod

Servings: 4 I Prep time: 10 minutes I Cook time: 1 hour and 30 minutes
Nutrition facts per serving: calories: 350; carbs: 3 gr; protein: 31 gr; fat: 6 gr.

Ingredients
- ✓ 2 cod fillets (about 350 gr for each)
- ✓ 1 orange
- ✓ 8 cherry tomatoes
- ✓ 8 green olives
- ✓ 1 tbsp of chopped parsley
- ✓ Olive oil, salt and pepper

Directions
- ➢ First, wash the cod fillets under cold running water, gut them and dab them with a paper towel to dry them.
- ➢ Then wash and cut the cherry tomatoes into pieces.
- ➢ Wash and chop a little parsley with a clove of garlic.
- ➢ Place a sheet of baking paper on the bottom of the ceramic pot.
- ➢ Brush the bottom and edges with a drizzle of oil, then lay the cod on them.
- ➢ At this point, in the belly of each cod fillet, place two slices of orange and 1 teaspoon of chopped parsley with garlic.
- ➢ Add the cherry tomatoes and chopped green olives around and on top of the cod.
- ➢ Season with salt and pepper, sprinkle everything with a large spoonful of chopped parsley and garlic, sprinkle with white wine and a spoonful of extra virgin olive oil.
- ➢ Lift the edges of the paper and pinch them together like sealing a cake. It doesn't have to be completely shut; don't be concerned if it doesn't stay still.
- ➢ Cover and cook on high for 1 hour and 30 minutes.
- ➢ After this time, check your fish, and if it is not done, keep on cooking for other 10 minutes.
- ➢ Serve your cod fillets immediately together with the vegetables and cooking juices.

Oat breaded squid rings

Servings: 4 I Prep time: 10 minutes I Cook time: 2 hours
Nutrition facts per serving: calories: 230; carbs: 4 gr; protein: 24 gr; fat: 3 gr.

Ingredients
- ✓ 500 gr of cleaned squid cut into rings
- ✓ 3 tbsp of oat flour
- ✓ 1 tbsp of olive oil
- ✓ 1 tbsp of mixed herbs
- ✓ Olive oil, salt and pepper

Directions
- ➢ First, finely chop the herbs
- ➢ Mix the chopped herbs with the oar flour, salt, and pepper.
- ➢ Season the squid with a tablespoon of oil and then mix with the oat flour mix.
- ➢ Pour all the ingredients into the slow cooker.
- ➢ Cook for 2 hours in high mode.
- ➢ Once this time has passed, you can serve your squid rings.

Olives and tomato sea bream

Servings: 4 I Prep time: 10 minutes I Cook time: 1 hour and 30 minutes
Nutrition facts per serving: calories: 350; carbs: 3 gr; protein: 31 gr; fat: 6 gr.

Ingredients
- ✓ 2 sea bream fillets (about 300 gr for each)
- ✓ 1 medium tomato

- ✓ 8 black olives
- ✓ 1 tbsp of salted capers
- ✓ ½ bunch of fresh parsley
- ✓ Olive oil, salt and pepper

Directions
- ➢ To cook the sea bream in the slow cooker you will need to prepare the various ingredients to put in the ceramic pot.
- ➢ First, wash the fish under cold running water, gut them and dab them with a paper towel to dry them.
- ➢ Then wash and cut the tomatoes into cubes, desalt the capers.
- ➢ Chop the parsley.
- ➢ At this point that you have all the ingredients ready, place a previously wet and squeezed piece of baking paper on the bottom of the ceramic pot.
- ➢ Brush the bottom and edges with a drizzle of oil, then lay the fish on them.
- ➢ At this point, in the belly of each sea bream, place two slices of lemon.
- ➢ Add the diced tomatoes, olives, and capers around and on top of the fish.
- ➢ Season with salt and pepper, sprinkle with parsley and ½ glass of white wine and a spoonful of extra virgin olive oil.
- ➢ Lift the edges of the paper and pinch them together like sealing a cake. It doesn't have to be completely shut; don't be concerned if it doesn't stay still. Cover and cook on high for 1 hour and 30 minutes. After this time, check your fish, it must be cooked but not flake too much.
- ➢ Serve your sea bream immediately together with the vegetables and cooking juices.

Orange and basil tuna

Servings: 4 I Prep time: 10 minutes I Cook time: 1 hour and 30 minutes
Nutrition facts per serving: calories: 380; carbs: 2 gr; protein: 36 gr; fat: 9 gr.

Ingredients
- ✓ 700 gr of tuna fillet
- ✓ 1 orange
- ✓ 1 tbsp of chopped basil
- ✓ 1 tbsp of chopped parsley
- ✓ Salt and pepper

Directions
- ➢ First, wash and remove the skin from the tuna.
- ➢ Then, wash and slice orange.
- ➢ Wash and chop both parsley and basil.
- ➢ Spread a sheet of parchment paper (or a liner) on the bottom of the pan.

- ➢ Place a few slices of orange on the bottom.
- ➢ Place the tuna on top of the lemon and season with salt and pepper to taste.
- ➢ Add basil and parsley and the remaining orange slices.
- ➢ Cook the tuna fillet with orange in low mode for an hour and a half.
- ➢ When fish is done, you can serve with orange slices.

Pine nuts and anchovy monkfish

Servings: 4 I Prep time: 10 minutes I Cook time: 3 hours
Nutrition facts per serving: calories: 340; carbs: 5 gr; protein: 31 gr; fat: 6 gr.

Ingredients
- ✓ 1 kg of monkfish fish
- ✓ 2 anchovy fillets
- ✓ 20 gr of pine nuts
- ✓ 1/2 carrot
- ✓ 3 tbsp of peeled tomato
- ✓ Olive oil, salt and pepper

Directions
- ➢ First, finely chop a piece of onion. Wash half a carrot and chop it.
- ➢ Wash a sprig of parsley too.
- ➢ In a pan, fry with a drizzle of olive oil, add the peeled and chopped tomato and the anchovy fillets.
- ➢ Pound the pine nuts and add them to the sauté.
- ➢ Wash, clean and cut the monkfish into pieces.
- ➢ Transfer everything to the slow cooker with the fish whole or in pieces, depending on the size.
- ➢ Add a glass of white wine, cover and cook on low for 3 hours.
- ➢ After three hours, remove the fish from the slow cooker and serve it hot directly on serving plates.

Rosemary and chilli baby octopus

Servings: 4 I Prep time: 10 minutes I Cook time: 3 hours
Nutrition facts per serving: calories: 340; carbs: 5 gr; protein: 31 gr; fat: 6 gr.

Ingredients
- ✓ 700 gr of baby octopus already cleaned
- ✓ 1 garlic clove
- ✓ 1 tbsp of chopped rosemary

- ✓ 1 tomato
- ✓ 1 chili pepper
- ✓ Olive oil and salt

Directions
- ➤ First clean the garlic, wash it, and chop it.
- ➤ Wash and dry tomato, then cut it into pieces.
- ➤ Chop finely chilli pepper.
- ➤ Clean and wash the octopus and let them dry.
- ➤ Then the fish in the slow cooker with the oil, garlic, rosemary, peeled tomatoes, and chilli.
- ➤ Close the lid and cook on low mode for 3 hours.
- ➤ Serve still hot with cooking juices.

Salmon with lemon dill and marjoram

Servings: 4 | Prep time: 10 minutes | Cook time: 1 hour and 30 minutes
Nutrition facts per serving: calories: 380; carbs: 2 gr; protein: 36 gr; fat: 9 gr.

Ingredients
- ✓ 700 gr of salmon fillet
- ✓ 1 lemon
- ✓ 1 tbsp of chopped marjoram
- ✓ 1 tbsp of chopped dill
- ✓ Olive oil, salt and pepper

Directions
- ➤ First, wash and remove the skin and bones from the salmon.
- ➤ Now, slice the lemon.
- ➤ Spread a sheet of parchment paper (or a liner) on the bottom of the pan.
- ➤ Place a few slices of lemon on the bottom.
- ➤ Place the salmon on top of the lemon and season with salt and pepper to taste.
- ➤ Add a few sprigs of marjoram and dill and the remaining lemon slices.
- ➤ A very important step to obtain a perfect result is to use the thermometer, in fact Cook times can vary according to the thickness of the fillet. If instead of a single fillet you have several slices available, it would be good that all are more or less of the same size, if not, put the thermometer in the larger piece.
- ➤ In any case, cook the salmon with lemon in low mode for an hour and a half, reaching a temperature of 56 ° c.
- ➤ When fish is done, you can serve with lemon slices.

Steamed squid

Servings: 4 | Prep time: 10 minutes | Cook time: 2 hours

Nutrition facts per serving: calories: 270; carbs: 7.7 gr; protein: 24 gr; fat: 5 gr.

Ingredients
- ✓ 750 gr of cleaned squid
- ✓ 200 gr of cherry tomatoes
- ✓ 1 glass of white wine
- ✓ 1 clove of garlic
- ✓ 1 small chilli
- ✓ Salt and pepper

Directions
- ➤ First, peel wash and mince the garlic and finely.
- ➤ Chop the chilli too.
- ➤ Put the garlic and chilli pepper on the bottom of the pot together with the tablespoon of oil.
- ➤ Wash and cut the cherry tomatoes into 4 wedges and put them in the pot, seasoning with a little salt and and pepper..
- ➤ Wash the squid well, cut the heads into rings and the tentacles into smaller pieces.
- ➤ Put the squid in the slow cooker and pour over the white wine.
- ➤ Mix everything quickly.
- ➤ Now move on to cooking stewed squid in the slow cooker.
- ➤ Set the slow cooker to high and cook for 2 hours.
- ➤ After two hours, remove the stewed squid and serve with the cooking sauce on serving plates.

Trout in herbs and tomatoes

Servings: 4 | Prep time: 10 minutes | Cook time: 1 hour and 30 minutes
Nutrition facts per serving: calories: 400; carbs: 6 gr; protein: 36 gr; fat: 9 gr.

Ingredients
- ✓ 700 gr of trout fillet
- ✓ 300 gr of peeled tomatoes
- ✓ 1 tbsp of chopped thyme
- ✓ 1 tbsp of chopped oregano
- ✓ Salt and pepper

Directions
- ➤ First, wash and remove the skin and bones from the trout fillet.
- ➤ Meanwhile, wash and chop both thyme and oregano.
- ➤ Spread a sheet of parchment paper (or a liner) on the bottom of the pan.
- ➤ Place the trout on top of the lemon and season with salt and pepper.
- ➤ Add peeled tomatoes.
- ➤ Add the herbs too.
- ➤ Now, you can cook your trout fillet in the slow cooker.

- ➤ Select low mode and cook trout for an hour and a half.
- ➤ When fish is done, you can serve with peeled tomatoes and cooking juices.

Soups and broths slow cooker recipes

Courgettes and tomato soup

Servings: 4 I Prep time: 10 minutes I Cook time: 14 hours
Nutrition facts per serving: calories: 310; carbs: 9 gr; protein: 4 gr; fat: 2 gr.

Ingredients
- ✓ 2 courgettes
- ✓ 200 gr of tomato puree
- ✓ 1 tbsp of powdered onion
- ✓ 1 tbsp of chopped parsley
- ✓ Salt and pepper

Directions
- ➤ First, peel wash and cut into cubes the 2 courgettes.
- ➤ Wash and chop parsley.
- ➤ Put courgettes and tomato puree in the slow cooker, put the water until it is lightly covered and then add powdered onion, salt, pepper and chopped parsley.
- ➤ Cook for 14 hours on low mode.
- ➤ When will be done you can serve it.

Cuttlefish and dried mushrooms soup

Servings: 4 I Prep time: 10 minutes I Cook time: 2 hours and 30 minutes
Nutrition facts per serving: calories: 230; carbs: 6 gr; protein: 22 gr; fat: 3 gr.

Ingredients
- ✓ 800 gr of cleaned cuttlefish
- ✓ 200 gr of tomato puree
- ✓ 2 cloves of garlic
- ✓ 2 tbsp dried mushrooms
- ✓ 2 tbsp of pine nuts

Directions
- ➤ First, soak the mushrooms in water and cut the cuttlefish into strips.
- ➤ Then, cut a little parsley finely, crush the garlic and take two anchovies in salt.

- ➤ Put everything in a pan with the hot oil and start making the sauté, melt the anchovies well and when the garlic is golden, remove it before it burns.
- ➤ At this point, add the cuttlefish and sauté them in the oil, when they are a little golden and then add the white wine.
- ➤ The cuttlefish will give a little water, let it go so that it can dry a little.
- ➤ Finally, put all the contents of the pan in the slow cooker, add the pine nuts, the drained and chopped mushrooms, the tomato puree and two tablespoons of concentrated tomato, add the water (preferably warm), until the cuttlefish is slightly covered.
- ➤ Salt lightly and turn on high for 2 and a half hours.
- ➤ At the end, season with salt and pepper.
- ➤ You can serve your cuttlefish soup.

Fish soup

Servings: 4 I Prep time: 10 minutes I Cook time: 3 hours
Nutrition facts per serving: calories: 180; carbs: 6 gr; protein: 16 gr; fat: 1 gr.

Ingredients
- ✓ 1 kg of cleaned mixed shellfish (mussels and clams)
- ✓ 2 cloves of garlic:
- ✓ 500 gr of tomatoes
- ✓ 1 tsp of chilli
- ✓ 2 tbsp of mixed salted aromatic herbs

Directions
- ➤ First of all, the fish must be cleaned and gutted before putting them in the slow cooker.
- ➤ After that, peel, wash and mince garlic into cubes, together with the chilli.
- ➤ Take the inner container of the slow cooker and allow the water to come out, placing it for about ten minutes on the flame over a not too high heat.
- ➤ Add the washed and chopped tomatoes and the aromatic herbs.
- ➤ It is then boiled for about 3 and a quarter hour.
- ➤ Fifteen minutes from the end, the clams, or bivalve molluscs we have chosen are added, so that they open and release their tasty water.
- ➤ In the end, everything is extracted from the slow cooker and served directly on the table, considering that everything will be very liquid due to the water released by the fish.
- ➤ Serve very hot.

Meat broth

Servings: 4 I Prep time: 10 minutes I Cook time: 8 hours
Nutrition facts per serving: calories: 200; carbs: 3 gr; protein: 14 gr; fat: 6 gr.

Ingredients
- ✓ 400 gr of meat for broth (such as pork ribs)
- ✓ 1 carrot
- ✓ 1 onion
- ✓ 1 stick of celery
- ✓ 2 litres of water
- ✓ Salt and pepper

Directions
- ➤ First, peel, wash, and chop together onion, celery, and carrot.
- ➤ Wash dry and put the meat, vegetables, pepper, and salt in the slow cooker.
- ➤ Then fill with water.
- ➤ Set the switch to low and let it go for 8 hours.
- ➤ At the end of cooking, filter the broth from the fat and impurities, and obviously nothing is thrown away, the meat and vegetables used can be set aside to eat or use it for other preparations.
- ➤ The broth is ready for being used.

Radicchio and blue cheese soup

Servings: 4 I Prep time: 10 minutes I Cook time: 2 hours
Nutrition facts per serving: calories: 190; carbs: 2 gr; protein: 16 gr; fat: 7 gr.

Ingredients
- ✓ 200 gr of radicchio leaves
- ✓ 300 gr of blue cheese
- ✓ 100 gr of grated parmesan cheese
- ✓ 1 teaspoon of smoked paprika
- ✓ 1 tbsp of mixed aromatic herbs

Directions
- ➤ First, wash the radicchio leaves well then chop.
- ➤ Cut the blue cheese into pieces.
- ➤ In the slow cooker pot add the blue cheese, the grated parmesan cheese, chopped radicchio, 1 tsp of onion powder, smoked paprika and the chopped aromatic herbs.
- ➤ Mix everything with a wooden ladle.
- ➤ Don't be afraid if the pot is full to the brim, everything will fall into place during cooking and the spinach will cook in the melted cheese.
- ➤ Cover and cook in low mode for 2 hours, stirring after the first hour of cooking and then finally after finishing the 2 hours.

- ➤ Serve your soup still hot.

Ragout soup

Servings: 4 I Prep time: 10 minutes I Cook time: 8/9 hours
Nutrition facts per serving: calories: 240; carbs: 3 gr; protein: 21 gr; fat: 10 gr.

Ingredients
- ✓ 400 gr minced meat
- ✓ 200 gr of pork sausage
- ✓ 1 litre of tomato sauce
- ✓ 2 carrots
- ✓ 1 glass of red wine

Directions
- ➤ Remove the sausage from the casing and add it to the meat.
- ➤ Peel a piece of onion and carrots, then chop them together.
- ➤ Then in a pan, brown the preparation for the ceiling, when ready, add the meat, stir, and brown it a little.
- ➤ Then blend with red wine.
- ➤ It will take about 10 - 15 minutes, wait for this fundamental moment because the meat is better flavoured, when the meat is ready, turn off the heat and put everything in the slow cooker.
- ➤ At this point you have to add only the tomato puree in order to cover a finger above the meat, finally season with salt and pepper.
- ➤ Now all that remains is to turn on the slow cooker in high mode and cook everything for 8 - 9 hours.
- ➤ Once 8 - 9 hours have passed, open the pot and serve your ragout soup.

Red wine beef soup

Servings: 4 I Prep time: 10 minutes I Cook time: 12 hours
Nutrition facts per serving: calories: 380; carbs: 3 gr, protein: 36 gr; fat: 7 gr.

Ingredients
- ✓ 800 gr of diced beef (better the muscle)
- ✓ 1 bottle of full-bodied red wine (it would take chianti)
- ✓ 2 cloves of garlic
- ✓ 1 tbsp black peppercorns
- ✓ Salt and pepper

Directions
- ➤ First clean the beef meat from excess of fat.
- ➤ Peel, wash and mince the garlic cloves.

➤ Put the meat, the crushed garlic, the pepper, and the wine into the slow cooker. The only precaution is that the wine must cover the meat.
➤ Turn on the slow cooker at low for 12 hours.
➤ When cooked, put the meat in a container and pour the sauce into a pan to make it shrink (you can use a little of oat flour).
➤ Add the reduced sauce to the meat again, mix well and serve your soup.

Spinach and cheese soup

Servings: 4 I Prep time: 10 minutes I Cook time: 2 hours
Nutrition facts per serving: calories: 190; carbs: 2 gr; protein: 16 gr; fat: 7 gr.

Ingredients
✓ 200 gr of brie cheese
✓ 200 gr of grated cheddar cheese
✓ 200 gr of fresh spinach leaves
✓ 1 teaspoon of garlic powder
✓ 1 tbsp of mixed aromatic herbs (rosemary, thyme, oregano, basil)

Directions
➤ First, wash the spinach leaves well and cut the brie into pieces.
➤ In the slow cooker pot add the brie cheese, the grated cheddar cheese, the spinach, the garlic powder, and the chopped aromatic herbs.
➤ Mix everything with a wooden ladle.
➤ Don't be afraid if the pot is full to the brim, everything will fall into place during cooking and the spinach will cook in the melted cheese.
➤ Cover and cook in low mode for 2 hours, stirring after the first hour of cooking and then finally after finishing the 2 hours.
➤ The soup is ready. Instead of turning off the slow cooker, set the warm mode.
➤ This will keep the cream at an ideal temperature until it's time to serve it.

Sweet and sour onion broth

Servings: 4 I Prep time: 10 minutes I Cook time: 3 hours
Nutrition facts per serving: calories: 70; carbs: 9 gr; protein: 1gr; fat: 0 gr.

Ingredients
✓ 600 gr of onions
✓ Half a glass of wine
✓ Half a glass of apple cider vinegar
✓ Half a glass of oil

✓ 40 gr of stevia powder
✓ Olive oil and salt

Directions
➤ First, you need to clean all the onions well and then place them inside the slow cooker pan.
➤ Over the onions, pour half a glass of wine, half a glass of vinegar, and half a glass of oil.
➤ Finally, add the stevia and mix everything.
➤ Cooking sweet and sour onions in the slow cooker.
➤ Cook for 3 hours on high. During this time, check the onions on a regular basis because the exact cooking time is dependent on their size. Eventually they should feel soft, but not flake off.
➤ The onions are now ready to eat or store in a jar after they have been cooked. If you want to serve them right away, brown them briefly in a pan.
➤ You can serve your onion broth.

Veggie broth

Servings: 4 I Prep time: 10 minutes I Cook time: 14 hours
Nutrition facts per serving: calories: 80; carbs: 8 gr; protein: 3 gr; fat: 0 gr.

Ingredients
✓ 2 courgettes
✓ 2 carrots
✓ 1 tbsp of smoked paprika
✓ 1 tbsp of chopped onion
✓ Water
✓ Salt and pepper

Directions
➤ First, peel wash and cut into cubes both courgettes and carrots.
➤ Put everything in the slow cooker, put the water until it is lightly covered and then add salt, paprika, and pepper.
➤ Cook for 14 hours on low mode.
➤ When veggies broth will be done you can serve it.

Velvety soup of leeks and carrots

Servings: 4 I Prep time: 10 minutes I Cook time: 2 hours and 30 minutes
Nutrition facts per serving: calories: 100; carbs: 8 gr; protein: 2 gr; fat: 3 gr.

Ingredients
✓ 500 g of carrots
✓ 2 leeks
✓ 1 clove of garlic

✓ 400 ml of water
✓ 1 tbsp of lemon juice
✓ Salt and pepper

Directions
➤ First peel and wash the carrots.
➤ Cut the carrots into pieces.
➤ Slice the leek by removing the outermost layer and the harder and too green parts, peel and chop the garlic.
➤ Fry the leeks and garlic in a pan with hot oil or directly in the slow cooker pan if it has a sauté function to fry.
➤ After a couple of minutes add the carrots and continue to fry for a few minutes another minute.
➤ Transfer the ingredients to the slow cooker (for those who have fried in a pan), cover with 400 ml of hot water.
➤ Set the cooking on high (or more) for 2 hours and 30 minutes.
➤ after the Cook time, when the carrots are very soft, we pass everything with an immersion blender (or possibly with a normal blender), add the salt, pepper, and lemon juice.
➤ if it seems too liquid, you can boil it for a few minutes and to restrict the excess liquids a little.
➤ Serve your soup still hot.

Walnut carrot and squid soup

Servings: 4 I Prep time: 10 minutes I Cook time: 2 hours and 30 minutes
Nutrition facts per serving: calories: 240; carbs: 9 gr; protein: 22 gr; fat: 3 gr.

Ingredients
✓ 800 gr of cleaned squid
✓ 200 gr of tomato puree
✓ 2 cloves of garlic
✓ 1 carrot
✓ 2 tbsp of walnuts

Directions
➤ First, peel and wash carrot, then cut into strips.
➤ Cut a little of chives finely and crush the garlic.
➤ Put everything in a pan with the hot oil and start making the sauté, and when the garlic is golden, remove it before it burns.
➤ At this point, add the squid and sauté them in the oil, when they are a little golden and then add a bit of white wine.
➤ Finally, put all the contents of the pan in the slow cooker, add the walnuts, and carrot.
➤ Add the water (preferably warm) and a bit tomato puree, until the squid is slightly covered.
➤ Salt lightly and turn on high for 2 and a half hours.

➤ At the end, season with salt and pepper.
➤ You can serve your squid and carrot soup.

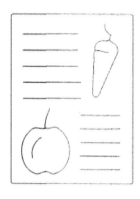

28 days meal plan

After showing you 5 ingredients very easy recipes, it's time to create meal plans. In this section, we will show you what to eat in four weeks for a perfect low-carb lifestyle.

Here you are some tips to follow this meal plans:
✓ Dinner and lunch can be interchanged, as well as snacks.
✓ You can drink 1 coffee a day and two cups of tea, strictly sugar-free.
✓ In this first phase of 4 weeks, carbs such as bread, pasta and rice are strictly prohibited.
✓ After these 4 weeks you can gradually add carbohydrates (first two weeks 30 g of bread, pasta or rice for lunch and dinner and then move on to 50 g in the following two weeks).

First week

MONDAY

Breakfast	A breakfast or a dessert of your choice from the recipes + a coffee or tea without sugar.
Morning snack	A snack, dessert (if you don't have it for breakfast or other snack) or a smoothie from recipes. Alternatively, either a greek yogurt or 30 gr of dried fruit.
Lunch	A plate of fish recipes of your choice + a plate of side dish recipes of your choice (or a green salad dressed with oil and apple cider vinegar)
Afternoon snack	A snack, dessert (if you don't have it for breakfast or other snack) or a smoothie from recipes. Alternatively, either a greek yogurt or 30 gr of dried fruit.
	A plate of beef recipes of

Dinner	your choice + a plate of side dish recipes of your choice (or a green salad dressed with oil and apple cider vinegar)

TUESDAY

Breakfast	A breakfast or a dessert of your choice from the recipes + a coffee or tea without sugar.
Morning snack	A snack, dessert (if you don't have it for breakfast or other snack) or a smoothie from recipes. Alternatively, either a greek yogurt or 30 gr of dried fruit.
Lunch	A plate of broth or soup + a plate of poultry or pork recipes
Afternoon snack	A snack, dessert (if you don't have it for breakfast or other snack) or a smoothie from recipes. Alternatively, either a greek yogurt or 30 gr of dried fruit.
Dinner	A dish of your choice of starters recipes + a dish of side dishes recipes (or alternatively a green salad dressed with oil and apple cider vinegar)

WEDNESDAY

Breakfast	A breakfast or a dessert of your choice from the recipes + a coffee or tea without sugar.
Morning snack	A snack, dessert (if you don't have it for breakfast or other snack) or a smoothie from recipes. Alternatively, either a greek yogurt or 30 gr of dried fruit.
Lunch	A plate of broth or soup + a plate of fish or starter recipes
Afternoon snack	A snack, dessert (if you don't have it for breakfast or other snack) or a smoothie from recipes.

	Alternatively, either a greek yogurt or 30 gr of dried fruit.
Dinner	A plate of fish recipes of your choice + a plate of side dish recipes of your choice (or a green salad dressed with oil and apple cider vinegar)

THURSDAY

Breakfast	A breakfast or a dessert of your choice from the recipes + a coffee or tea without sugar.
Morning snack	A snack, dessert (if you don't have it for breakfast or other snack) or a smoothie from recipes. Alternatively, either a greek yogurt or 30 gr of dried fruit.
Lunch	A plate of beef recipes of your choice + a plate of side dish recipes of your choice (or a green salad dressed with oil and apple cider vinegar)
Afternoon snack	A snack, dessert (if you don't have it for breakfast or other snack) or a smoothie from recipes. Alternatively, either a greek yogurt or 30 gr of dried fruit.
Dinner	A plate of broth or soup + a plate of poultry or pork recipes

FRIDAY

Breakfast	A breakfast or a dessert of your choice from the recipes + a coffee or tea without sugar.
Morning snack	A snack, dessert (if you don't have it for breakfast or other snack) or a smoothie from recipes. Alternatively, either a greek yogurt or 30 gr of dried fruit.
Lunch	A dish of your choice of starters recipes + a dish of side dishes recipes (or

	alternatively a green salad dressed with oil and apple cider vinegar)
Afternoon snack	A snack, dessert (if you don't have it for breakfast or other snack) or a smoothie from recipes. Alternatively, either a greek yogurt or 30 gr of dried fruit.
Dinner	A plate of fish recipes of your choice + a plate of side dish recipes of your choice (or a green salad dressed with oil and apple cider vinegar)

SATURDAY

Breakfast	A breakfast or a dessert of your choice from the recipes + a coffee or tea without sugar.
Morning snack	A snack, dessert (if you don't have it for breakfast or other snack) or a smoothie from recipes. Alternatively, either a greek yogurt or 30 gr of dried fruit.
Lunch	A dish of your choice of starters recipes + a dish of fish recipes
Afternoon snack	A snack, dessert (if you don't have it for breakfast or other snack) or a smoothie from recipes. Alternatively, either a greek yogurt or 30 gr of dried fruit.
Dinner	A plate of broth or soup + a plate of fish recipes

SUNDAY

Breakfast	A breakfast or a dessert of your choice from the recipes + a coffee or tea without sugar.
Morning snack	A snack, dessert (if you don't have it for breakfast or other snack) or a smoothie from recipes. Alternatively, either a greek yogurt or 30 gr of dried fruit.
	A dish of your choice of

Lunch	starters recipes + a dish of meat recipes.
Afternoon snack	A snack, dessert (if you don't have it for breakfast or other snack) or a smoothie from recipes. Alternatively, either a greek yogurt or 30 gr of dried fruit.
Dinner	A plate of fish recipes of your choice + a plate of side dish recipes of your choice (or a green salad dressed with oil and apple cider vinegar)

Second week

MONDAY

Breakfast	A breakfast or a dessert of your choice from the recipes + a coffee or tea without sugar.
Morning snack	A snack, dessert (if you don't have it for breakfast or other snack) or a smoothie from recipes. Alternatively, either a greek yogurt or 30 gr of dried fruit.
Lunch	A plate of fish recipes of your choice + a plate of side dish recipes of your choice (or a green salad dressed with oil and apple cider vinegar)
Afternoon snack	A snack, dessert (if you don't have it for breakfast or other snack) or a smoothie from recipes. Alternatively, either a greek yogurt or 30 gr of dried fruit.
Dinner	A plate of beef recipes of your choice + a plate of side dish recipes of your choice (or a green salad dressed with oil and apple cider vinegar)

TUESDAY

Breakfast	A breakfast or a dessert of your choice from the recipes + a coffee or tea without sugar.

Morning snack	A snack, dessert (if you don't have it for breakfast or other snack) or a smoothie from recipes. Alternatively, either a greek yogurt or 30 gr of dried fruit.
Lunch	A plate of broth or soup + a plate of poultry or pork recipes
Afternoon snack	A snack, dessert (if you don't have it for breakfast or other snack) or a smoothie from recipes. Alternatively, either a greek yogurt or 30 gr of dried fruit.
Dinner	A dish of your choice of starters recipes + a dish of side dishes recipes (or alternatively a green salad dressed with oil and apple cider vinegar)

WEDNESDAY

Breakfast	A breakfast or a dessert of your choice from the recipes + a coffee or tea without sugar.
Morning snack	A snack, dessert (if you don't have it for breakfast or other snack) or a smoothie from recipes. Alternatively, either a greek yogurt or 30 gr of dried fruit.
Lunch	A plate of broth or soup + a plate of fish or starter recipes
Afternoon snack	A snack, dessert (if you don't have it for breakfast or other snack) or a smoothie from recipes. Alternatively, either a greek yogurt or 30 gr of dried fruit.
Dinner	A plate of fish recipes of your choice + a plate of side dish recipes of your choice (or a green salad dressed with oil and apple cider vinegar)

THURSDAY

	A breakfast or a dessert of

Breakfast	your choice from the recipes + a coffee or tea without sugar.
Morning snack	A snack, dessert (if you don't have it for breakfast or other snack) or a smoothie from recipes. Alternatively, either a greek yogurt or 30 gr of dried fruit.
Lunch	A plate of beef recipes of your choice + a plate of side dish recipes of your choice (or a green salad dressed with oil and apple cider vinegar)
Afternoon snack	A snack, dessert (if you don't have it for breakfast or other snack) or a smoothie from recipes. Alternatively, either a greek yogurt or 30 gr of dried fruit.
Dinner	A plate of broth or soup + a plate of poultry or pork recipes

FRIDAY

Breakfast	A breakfast or a dessert of your choice from the recipes + a coffee or tea without sugar.
Morning snack	A snack, dessert (if you don't have it for breakfast or other snack) or a smoothie from recipes. Alternatively, either a greek yogurt or 30 gr of dried fruit.
Lunch	A dish of your choice of starters recipes + a dish of side dishes recipes (or alternatively a green salad dressed with oil and apple cider vinegar)
Afternoon snack	A snack, dessert (if you don't have it for breakfast or other snack) or a smoothie from recipes. Alternatively, either a greek yogurt or 30 gr of dried fruit.
Dinner	A plate of fish recipes of your choice + a plate of side dish recipes of your

	choice (or a green salad dressed with oil and apple cider vinegar)

SATURDAY

Breakfast	A breakfast or a dessert of your choice from the recipes + a coffee or tea without sugar.
Morning snack	A snack, dessert (if you don't have it for breakfast or other snack) or a smoothie from recipes. Alternatively, either a greek yogurt or 30 gr of dried fruit.
Lunch	A dish of your choice of starters recipes + a dish of fish recipes
Afternoon snack	A snack, dessert (if you don't have it for breakfast or other snack) or a smoothie from recipes. Alternatively, either a greek yogurt or 30 gr of dried fruit.
Dinner	A plate of broth or soup + a plate of fish recipes

SUNDAY

Breakfast	A breakfast or a dessert of your choice from the recipes + a coffee or tea without sugar.
Morning snack	A snack, dessert (if you don't have it for breakfast or other snack) or a smoothie from recipes. Alternatively, either a greek yogurt or 30 gr of dried fruit.
Lunch	A dish of your choice of starters recipes + a dish of meat recipes
Afternoon snack	A snack, dessert (if you don't have it for breakfast or other snack) or a smoothie from recipes. Alternatively, either a greek yogurt or 30 gr of dried fruit.
Dinner	A plate of fish recipes of your choice + a plate of side dish recipes of your choice (or a green salad

	dressed with oil and apple cider vinegar)

Third week

MONDAY

Breakfast	A breakfast or a dessert of your choice from the recipes + a coffee or tea without sugar.
Morning snack	A snack, dessert (if you don't have it for breakfast or other snack) or a smoothie from recipes. Alternatively, either a greek yogurt or 30 gr of dried fruit.
Lunch	A plate of fish recipes of your choice + a plate of side dish recipes of your choice (or a green salad dressed with oil and apple cider vinegar)
Afternoon snack	A snack, dessert (if you don't have it for breakfast or other snack) or a smoothie from recipes. Alternatively, either a greek yogurt or 30 gr of dried fruit.
Dinner	A plate of beef recipes of your choice + a plate of side dish recipes of your choice (or a green salad dressed with oil and apple cider vinegar)

TUESDAY

Breakfast	A breakfast or a dessert of your choice from the recipes + a coffee or tea without sugar.
Morning snack	A snack, dessert (if you don't have it for breakfast or other snack) or a smoothie from recipes. Alternatively, either a greek yogurt or 30 gr of dried fruit.
Lunch	A plate of broth or soup + a plate of poultry or pork recipes
Afternoon snack	A snack, dessert (if you don't have it for breakfast or other snack) or a smoothie from recipes.

	Alternatively, either a greek yogurt or 30 gr of dried fruit.
Dinner	A dish of your choice of starters recipes + a dish of side dishes recipes (or alternatively a green salad dressed with oil and apple cider vinegar)

WEDNESDAY

Breakfast	A breakfast or a dessert of your choice from the recipes + a coffee or tea without sugar.
Morning snack	A snack, dessert (if you don't have it for breakfast or other snack) or a smoothie from recipes. Alternatively, either a greek yogurt or 30 gr of dried fruit.
Lunch	A plate of broth or soup + a plate of fish or starter recipes
Afternoon snack	A snack, dessert (if you don't have it for breakfast or other snack) or a smoothie from recipes. Alternatively, either a greek yogurt or 30 gr of dried fruit.
Dinner	A plate of fish recipes of your choice + a plate of side dish recipes of your choice (or a green salad dressed with oil and apple cider vinegar)

THURSDAY

Breakfast	A breakfast or a dessert of your choice from the recipes + a coffee or tea without sugar.
Morning snack	A snack, dessert (if you don't have it for breakfast or other snack) or a smoothie from recipes. Alternatively, either a greek yogurt or 30 gr of dried fruit.
Lunch	A plate of beef recipes of your choice + a plate of side dish recipes of your choice (or a green salad

	dressed with oil and apple cider vinegar)
Afternoon snack	A snack, dessert (if you don't have it for breakfast or other snack) or a smoothie from recipes. Alternatively, either a greek yogurt or 30 gr of dried fruit.
Dinner	A plate of broth or soup + a plate of poultry or pork recipes

FRIDAY

Breakfast	A breakfast or a dessert of your choice from the recipes + a coffee or tea without sugar.
Morning snack	A snack, dessert (if you don't have it for breakfast or other snack) or a smoothie from recipes. Alternatively, either a greek yogurt or 30 gr of dried fruit.
Lunch	A dish of your choice of starters recipes + a dish of side dishes recipes (or alternatively a green salad dressed with oil and apple cider vinegar)
Afternoon snack	A snack, dessert (if you don't have it for breakfast or other snack) or a smoothie from recipes. Alternatively, either a greek yogurt or 30 gr of dried fruit.
Dinner	A plate of fish recipes of your choice + a plate of side dish recipes of your choice (or a green salad dressed with oil and apple cider vinegar)

SATURDAY

Breakfast	A breakfast or a dessert of your choice from the recipes + a coffee or tea without sugar.
Morning snack	A snack, dessert (if you don't have it for breakfast or other snack) or a smoothie from recipes. Alternatively, either a

	greek yogurt or 30 gr of dried fruit.
Lunch	A plate of poultry or pork recipes of your choice + a plate of side dish recipes of your choice (or a green salad dressed with oil and apple cider vinegar)
Afternoon snack	A snack, dessert (if you don't have it for breakfast or other snack) or a smoothie from recipes. Alternatively, either a greek yogurt or 30 gr of dried fruit.
Dinner	A plate of broth or soup + a plate of fish recipes

SUNDAY

Breakfast	A breakfast or a dessert of your choice from the recipes + a coffee or tea without sugar.
Morning snack	A snack, dessert (if you don't have it for breakfast or other snack) or a smoothie from recipes. Alternatively, either a greek yogurt or 30 gr of dried fruit.
Lunch	A dish of your choice of starters recipes + a dish of meat recipes.
Afternoon snack	A snack, dessert (if you don't have it for breakfast or other snack) or a smoothie from recipes. Alternatively, either a greek yogurt or 30 gr of dried fruit.
Dinner	A plate of fish recipes of your choice + a plate of side dish recipes of your choice (or a green salad dressed with oil and apple cider vinegar)

Fourth week

MONDAY

Breakfast	A breakfast or a dessert of your choice from the recipes + a coffee or tea without sugar.
	A snack, dessert (if you

Morning snack	don't have it for breakfast or other snack) or a smoothie from recipes. Alternatively, either a greek yogurt or 30 gr of dried fruit.
Lunch	A plate of fish recipes of your choice + a plate of side dish recipes of your choice (or a green salad dressed with oil and apple cider vinegar)
Afternoon snack	A snack, dessert (if you don't have it for breakfast or other snack) or a smoothie from recipes. Alternatively, either a greek yogurt or 30 gr of dried fruit.
Dinner	A plate of beef recipes of your choice + a plate of side dish recipes of your choice (or a green salad dressed with oil and apple cider vinegar)

TUESDAY

Breakfast	A breakfast or a dessert of your choice from the recipes + a coffee or tea without sugar.
Morning snack	A snack, dessert (if you don't have it for breakfast or other snack) or a smoothie from recipes. Alternatively, either a greek yogurt or 30 gr of dried fruit.
Lunch	A plate of broth or soup + a plate of poultry or pork recipes
Afternoon snack	A snack, dessert (if you don't have it for breakfast or other snack) or a smoothie from recipes. Alternatively, either a greek yogurt or 30 gr of dried fruit.
Dinner	A dish of your choice of starters recipes + a dish of side dishes recipes (or alternatively a green salad dressed with oil and apple cider vinegar)

WEDNESDAY

Breakfast	A breakfast or a dessert of your choice from the recipes + a coffee or tea without sugar.
Morning snack	A snack, dessert (if you don't have it for breakfast or other snack) or a smoothie from recipes. Alternatively, either a greek yogurt or 30 gr of dried fruit.
Lunch	A plate of broth or soup + a plate of fish or starter recipes
Afternoon snack	A snack, dessert (if you don't have it for breakfast or other snack) or a smoothie from recipes. Alternatively, either a greek yogurt or 30 gr of dried fruit.
Dinner	A plate of fish recipes of your choice + a plate of side dish recipes of your choice (or a green salad dressed with oil and apple cider vinegar)

THURSDAY

Breakfast	A breakfast or a dessert of your choice from the recipes + a coffee or tea without sugar.
Morning snack	A snack, dessert (if you don't have it for breakfast or other snack) or a smoothie from recipes. Alternatively, either a greek yogurt or 30 gr of dried fruit.
Lunch	A plate of beef recipes of your choice + a plate of side dish recipes of your choice (or a green salad dressed with oil and apple cider vinegar)
Afternoon snack	A snack, dessert (if you don't have it for breakfast or other snack) or a smoothie from recipes. Alternatively, either a greek yogurt or 30 gr of dried fruit.
Dinner	A plate of broth or soup + a plate of poultry or pork

	recipes

FRIDAY

Breakfast	A breakfast or a dessert of your choice from the recipes + a coffee or tea without sugar.
Morning snack	A snack, dessert (if you don't have it for breakfast or other snack) or a smoothie from recipes. Alternatively, either a greek yogurt or 30 gr of dried fruit.
Lunch	A dish of your choice of starters recipes + a dish of side dishes recipes (or alternatively a green salad dressed with oil and apple cider vinegar)
Afternoon snack	A snack, dessert (if you don't have it for breakfast or other snack) or a smoothie from recipes. Alternatively, either a greek yogurt or 30 gr of dried fruit.
Dinner	A plate of fish recipes of your choice + a plate of side dish recipes of your choice (or a green salad dressed with oil and apple cider vinegar)

SATURDAY

Breakfast	A breakfast or a dessert of your choice from the recipes + a coffee or tea without sugar.
Morning snack	A snack, dessert (if you don't have it for breakfast or other snack) or a smoothie from recipes. Alternatively, either a greek yogurt or 30 gr of dried fruit.
Lunch	A plate of poultry or pork recipes of your choice + a plate of side dish recipes of your choice (or a green salad dressed with oil and apple cider vinegar)
Afternoon snack	A snack, dessert (if you don't have it for breakfast or other snack) or a

	smoothie from recipes. Alternatively, either a greek yogurt or 30 gr of dried fruit.
Dinner	A plate of broth or soup + a plate of fish recipes

SUNDAY

Breakfast	A breakfast or a dessert of your choice from the recipes + a coffee or tea without sugar.
Morning snack	A snack, dessert (if you don't have it for breakfast or other snack) or a smoothie from recipes. Alternatively, either a greek yogurt or 30 gr of dried fruit.
Lunch	A dish of your choice of starters recipes + a dish of meat recipes
Afternoon snack	A snack, dessert (if you don't have it for breakfast or other snack) or a smoothie from recipes. Alternatively, either a greek yogurt or 30 gr of dried fruit.
Dinner	A plate of fish recipes of your choice + a plate of side dish recipes of your choice (or a green salad dressed with oil and apple cider vinegar)

Printed in Great Britain
by Amazon

11931089R00072